Praise for *Implementing Value-Based Healthcare* by Sally Lewis

'Sally Lewis has given us an essential history of value-based healthcare mindset and method, and a pragmatic guidebook for local, national and global healthcare transformation. Through examples and frank assessment of the hard work required, she reminds us that getting to the summit of value is a team effort, and our compass must ever be the health outcomes important to patients.'

> — **Jennifer Bright**, president and CEO of the International Consortium for Health Outcomes Measurement (ICHOM)

'*Implementing Value-Based Healthcare* is essential reading for anyone shaping the future of healthcare. With clarity and insight, Sally Lewis distils the hard-won lessons and the challenges and rewards of implementing value-based healthcare, from frontline practice to system-wide change.'

> — **Dr Jonathan Broomberg**, group deputy CEO at Vitality and non-executive director at the UCLH Foundation Trust

'As a dedicated physician operating within a healthcare system that does not deliver on its mission, Sally Lewis channels her personal experience and frustration into a book that provides actionable strategies for others who, like her, choose not to throw their hands up in the air but to lead change from within. Lewis's journey shows us that there are many great challenges to overcome and that improving healthcare is not for the faint of heart. But as *Implementing Value-Based Healthcare* makes clear, there is also hope, and many people who will help you along the way.'

> — **Susanna Gallani**, Tai Family Associate Professor of Business Administration, Harvard Business School

'The last twenty years have been dominated by the quality paradigm: the belief that all that was needed was for healthcare managers and clinicians to increase the quality, safety and efficiency of clinical care for patients. However, it is now clear that unless we measure outcome as well as quality and relate the use of resources to populations as well as patients, universal healthcare is unsustainable. This means that value-based healthcare is now the dominant paradigm. Sally Lewis has brought about the required paradigm shift in Wales. What she has done is a very good example of what the leaders and managers of health services for populations need to do. The key is to find and support people like Lewis because strong leadership is needed to change the culture. This book summarizes her journey clearly and provides an evidence-based resource for people in leadership positions globally.'

— **Professor Sir Muir Gray,** executive director of the Oxford Value and Stewardship Programme, director of the Optimal Ageing Programme, and founding director of the Critical Appraisal Skills Programme (CASP)

'Sally Lewis has written a powerful and practical guide to one of the most urgent challenges in healthcare today. Drawing on real-world lessons from Wales and beyond, she shows how value-based healthcare can improve patient outcomes while also making systems more sustainable. A must-read for clinicians, policymakers and leaders seeking a path to better health outcomes for individuals and communities.'

— **Professor Zoe Wainer,** Deputy Secretary, Community & Public Health at Victorian Department of Health

Implementing Value-Based Healthcare

PERSPECTIVES

Series editor: Professor Diane Coyle

The BRIC Road to Growth — Jim O'Neill

Reinventing London — Bridget Rosewell

Rediscovering Growth: After the Crisis — Andrew Sentance

Why Fight Poverty? — Julia Unwin

Identity Is The New Money — David Birch

Housing: Where's the Plan? — Kate Barker

Bad Habits, Hard Choices: Using the Tax System to Make Us Healthier — David Fell

A Better Politics: How Government Can Make Us Happier — Danny Dorling

Are Trams Socialist? Why Britain Has No Transport Policy — Christian Wolmar

Travel Fast or Smart? A Manifesto for an Intelligent Transport Policy — David Metz

Britain's Cities, Britain's Future — Mike Emmerich

Before Babylon, Beyond Bitcoin: From Money That We Understand To Money That Understands Us — David Birch

The Weaponization of Trade: The Great Unbalancing of Politics and Economics — Rebecca Harding and Jack Harding

Driverless Cars: On a Road to Nowhere? — Christian Wolmar

Digital Transformation at Scale: Why the Strategy Is Delivery — Andrew Greenway, Ben Terrett, Mike Bracken and Tom Loosemore

Gaming Trade: Win–Win Strategies for the Digital Era — Rebecca Harding and Jack Harding

The Currency Cold War: Cash and Cryptography, Hash Rates and Hegemony — David Birch

Catastrophe and Systemic Change: Learning from the Grenfell Tower Fire and Other Disasters — Gill Kernick

Transport for Humans: Are We Nearly There Yet? — Pete Dyson and Rory Sutherland

Technology Is Not Neutral: A Short Guide to Technology Ethics — Stephanie Hare

Good To Go? Decarbonising Travel After the Pandemic — David Metz

The World at Economic War: How to Rebuild Security in a Weaponized Global Economy — Rebecca Harding

Implementing Value-Based Healthcare: An Insider's Guide to Improving Patient Outcomes and Creating Sustainable Systems — Sally Lewis

Implementing Value-Based Healthcare

An Insider's Guide to Improving
Patient Outcomes and
Creating Sustainable Systems

Sally Lewis

LONDON PUBLISHING PARTNERSHIP

Published by London Publishing Partnership
www.londonpublishingpartnership.co.uk

Published in association with
Enlightenment Economics
www.enlightenmenteconomics.com

ISBN: 978-1-916749-51-1 (pbk)
ISBN: 978-1-916749-52-8 (iPDF)
ISBN: 978-1-916749-53-5 (epub)

A catalogue record for this book is
available from the British Library

This book has been composed in Candara

Copy-edited and typeset by
T&T Productions Ltd, London
www.tandtproductions.com

Printed and bound in Great Britain
by Hobbs the Printers Ltd

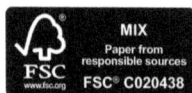

For Robbie, Maya, Tilly and Georgie

Contents

Foreword by Dr Stefan Larsson　　　　　　　　　　xi

Moral injury: why we must tackle the global crisis in
healthcare　　　　　　　　　　　　　　　　　　xix

Acknowledgements　　　　　　　　　　　　　　xxv

PART I
A STORY OF VALUE-BASED HEALTHCARE IN PRACTICE　1

CHAPTER 1
Beginnings: the roots of value-based healthcare
in Wales and beyond　　　　　　　　　　　　　3

CHAPTER 2
Velvet bulldozers: getting vaue-based healthcare
off the ground　　　　　　　　　　　　　　　29

CHAPTER 3
A gentle revolution from within　　　　　　　　53

PART II
HOW TO DRIVE VALUE FOR POPULATIONS, PATHWAYS AND PEOPLE　77

CHAPTER 4
A person is not a disease: achieving better outcomes
for people　　　　　　　　　　　　　　　　　83

CHAPTER 5
Making a difference: driving value aross pathways
of care   103

CHAPTER 6
True north: driving value for populations   129

PART III
LESSONS ON INFRASTRUCTURE   149

CHAPTER 7
Turning data into wisdom: the foundation of
value-based decisions   151

CHAPTER 8
Passing the baton: what next for value-based
healthcare?   189

About the author   199

Notes   201

Foreword

When I was asked by Professor Lewis to write this foreword, I was honoured and thrilled to do so. Having observed and learned from her work for more than a decade, I was really excited to be one of the first to read the full story. However, as I engaged in actually writing this text, my daughter was in the final weeks of her pregnancy and about to deliver my wife's and my first grandchild.

After a demanding first pregnancy, during which a premature delivery was very close, our granddaughter Ester was born eight days late. All went well. Although our daughter and her husband are socioeconomically advantaged and their parents well-connected, the excellent support given throughout the pregnancy and delivery was supplied by the public healthcare system in southern Stockholm – care that is available to all the country's citizens.

One of the characteristics of our most civilized societies has to be the good health and long life expectancy of their citizens. Good health ensures that as many as possible can flourish and contribute their capabilities and talents to the progress and prosperity of their society. Human reproductive biology and the rapid evolution of our societies limit our ability to predict which talents or capabilities will be particularly valuable in the future. Consequently, every ambitious civilized society must have health equity as one of its priorities.

Health systems are complex and adaptive. As with any evolutionary process, health system progress cannot be forced top down, but emerges bottom up, enabled and guided by a favourable ecosystem. A couple of the enablers of such a health ecosystem are an educational system that identifies and develops talent, and provision of a good basic education that includes health literacy for all. Another is free academic institutions that can research and explore the frontiers of human knowledge about health and disease. A society that promotes entrepreneurship and facilitates industrial development is a requirement if meaningful innovations and useful tools are to be available to patients and caregivers at low costs. We also need adequate investment to back the infrastructure and people that support health maintenance and treatment of those who are not well. We must establish funding models that secure universal access to prevention and appropriate care and thoughtful stewardship of our resources. And finally, we need a legal and regulatory framework that secures all of the above while meeting the need for continuous change.

At a high level, the public health of a country can be defined in several ways. Two often-used measures are quality-adjusted life years (QALYs) and healthy life years (HLYs). Nations that typically end up at the top of such rankings are the Scandinavian countries, Switzerland, Australia and Japan. These nations have addressed the critical enablers above, although they would all recognize there is still ample room for improvement.

However, in these nations as in the rest of the world, healthcare systems are facing a growing crisis that consists, arguably, of three parts: value, evidence and purpose. The value of many of our investments is questionable as costs are outgrowing public health improvements; because current research priorities limit the evidence required for effective clinical decision making; and, finally, because the growing focus on process optimization, production volumes and clinical efficiency is leading to stress-related disease and a people crisis among care providers. Increasingly, the sustainability of our health systems is questioned worldwide.

One of the most dramatic consequences of the industrial and scientific revolutions has been the improvements in public health. But healthcare has also become increasingly complex and fragmented, and there is growing recognition that we need to transform how systems are managed. In the 1920s Dr Ernst Codman challenged his colleagues at Massachusetts General Hospital in Boston, stressing the importance of the quality of the care provided and arguing that this must be defined by an institution's ability to deliver measurably superior health outcomes for its patients. In the 1960s Avedis Donabedian stated that the ultimate measure of healthcare quality should be the outcomes for patients. Later, Sir Muir Gray and others built and elaborated on this argument, but it was not until work by Elizabeth Teisberg and Michael Porter during the first years of the twenty-first century that value-based healthcare was defined as the ultimate way to redefine the healthcare systems of the future.

Important innovations and numerous useful tools have been established in the past 15 years, contributing to tremendous progress in transforming our healthcare systems to become more patient-centric and outcomes-focused. The number of research papers on topics related to value-based healthcare has grown exponentially in the past decade and a half, and several important books have been published to describe the progress through insightful case studies and clever frameworks, extracting learnings for others to build on. However, most of the latter work has been published by academics, management consultants or multinational organizations such as the World Economic Forum or the OECD. Until now, that is.

We should be grateful that Professor Lewis has now written this excellent book. It is the first of its kind: written by someone who has had a critical role in health system transformation, from the very first ideas and attempts to test value-based healthcare in local pilots to a situation today where national leaders in Wales claim that 'value-based healthcare has become business as usual'. She has led work from the bottom to the top of the pyramid and has been more willing than most to get her hands dirty. She illustrates the day-to-day challenges, the time and commitment that are needed, the necessary multidisciplinary collaboration and the senior leadership support that is required. Professor Lewis summarizes her experiences, learnings and insights in a very personal, clear and convincing way.

Throughout the book Lewis argues how critical it is for the improvement of healthcare that we are data and evidence based. However, while clinicians today are drowning in data, she makes the important point that they are starved of actionable information that can facilitate decisions to improve patient care. She argues that we must focus on what matters for patients: 'In essence it is only by capturing and understanding clinical and patient-reported outcomes that we can make a judgment about whether we are getting care right.'

It is essential when seeking to understand outcomes that matter to patients that we systematically ask for patient input. Although Lewis emphasizes that outcomes that matter to patients will inevitably have to be a mixture of input from clinicians, patients and others, 'the new kid on the block', as she puts it, is patient-reported outcome measures (PROMs). The book provides a rich description of the introduction and use of PROMs in Wales, detailing the challenges for data capture and integration into electronic medical records, how PROMs are used in clinical practice, and ultimately how this data has the potential to change clinical behaviours and culture.

Professor Lewis book also provides a thoughtful practitioner's perspective on value-based healthcare in general. She argues that value-based healthcare should not be seen as a threat to other good initiatives to increase productivity or improve the quality of our healthcare systems. Instead, it is a unifying theme and logic to establish common ground and shared goals across many of the various initiatives that have been launched over the past decades. One example is her discussion on 'person-centred care'. Some have argued that this is different from value-based healthcare, but Lewis instead states that personalized care is precisely what value-based healthcare wants to achieve. She describes how value-based healthcare offers the data and frameworks that are needed for clinical teams to strengthen their effort to deliver care adapted to individual needs and, ultimately, what some call 'the art of medicine'.

Lewis, who has worked with value-based healthcare across Wales, has the unique experience required to provide a powerful system-wide perspective on the changes that are needed. She makes clear that outcome data, although critical, is not enough. Access to data needs to be backed by incentives and rational payment models, by well-designed IT systems to facilitate secure data sharing and translation of data to insights for decision making, and by reconfiguration of care with collaboration along the care pathways. A wonderful example she shares is from maternity care in Kenya delivered by MomCare, illustrating the difference between traditional 'quality improvement' and the continuous improvement of patient value. Another important discussion is on the differences between today's methodology of health technology assessments in the adoption of new industry products and the essential role that value-based healthcare and outcomes measurement should play to ensure that new products de facto deliver on their promise in the real world.

Another of the book's strong points is explaining the universality of value-based healthcare. With its focus on patient populations defined by risk, a clinical condition or a combination of conditions, the outcomes that patients aspire to are the same irrespective of where in the world they live or come from. Value-based healthcare is therefore a platform for international collaboration and learning, and Wales has been an important part of this international community since the early days of Professor Lewis's work.

A point that is not so often discussed in value-based healthcare is the importance of educating and engaging the public in the changes towards high-value care. As others have done, Lewis makes the point that we must build our efforts on patient input and insights, but also, in doing so, she argues that we must mobilize the patient community (and voters) to influence policy-makers. In today's political landscape this is critical in countries where rhetoric and bipartisan polarization risk the longer-term continuity and rationality of necessary healthcare reforms.

An important theme of the book is multidisciplinary collaboration. As Professor Lewis states: 'None of us as individuals, and no single profession, can achieve radical healthcare transformation alone. We must work it out together or we will fail apart.' She argues that establishing trust across professional boundaries is key and that this is particularly important among respected senior clinical colleagues, who can embrace the new ways of working or resist the changes.

Lewis shares many examples of multidisciplinary teams she has worked with, each member bringing important and complementary expertise to the work. One example is outcomes-measurement expertise, which is crucial given the central role of this data. She praises the PROMs team she worked with, and more broadly she argues for the importance of having colleagues reliably handling the scientific complexity of validating outcomes measurement, risk adjustments and the proper interpretation of the data. Similarly, it is important to make sure that you have the right competence on the team to analyse costs and resources used along the care pathways.

I really like the warm and rich profiles Professor Lewis has written of some of the key expert leaders she has worked with during Wales's value-based healthcare programme. They illustrate the complementary nature of capabilities, as well as the shared purpose and the willingness to collaborate to put patients first. It is clear that it takes a village.

Just as multidisciplinary collaboration is a key theme in the book, another is the importance of visionary and bold leadership. Lewis clearly feels she has been very fortunate in the trust and mandate given to her by many senior leaders over the years: 'We were allowed to proceed with a degree of uncertainty that would not normally have been entertained. We were given freedom to act and we were allowed to fail.' She later adds: 'This early freedom to act was a critical factor in the subsequent momentum for value-based healthcare in Wales.'

With senior leaders on board, the Welsh example also illustrates a number of other change-management conditions that have been critical to progress. Professor Lewis shares a rich section on the importance of cultural change, and stresses that, ultimately, value-based healthcare requires substantial changes in behaviours across healthcare systems. This is a chicken and egg question, but arguably behaviours are in most cases rational, so the changes in culture require outcomes data, transparency, incentives, organizational structure and so on that promote the desired behaviours.

One lever for cultural change that the book discusses is education. Lewis describes her very positive experiences from joint educational programmes bringing together multidisciplinary participants: clinicians, managers, financial experts, informaticians, etc.

Another positive experience described in the book is the establishment of a forum for national coordination and the sharing of experiences: specifically, the National Value-Based Healthcare Delivery Group. For those familiar with the reform programme in the Netherlands, this initiative resembles the Linnean Group established over a decade ago to bring together the stakeholders across the Netherlands to discuss value-based healthcare and align on both priorities and the direction of travel.

Finally, change is hard in any organization, and change within healthcare organizations can be particularly challenging. Any ambitious change programme will be challenged – at times, even disrupted. Professor Lewis describes the disruption of the Welsh value-based healthcare programme by the Covid-19 pandemic. The entire effort was shut down for 18 months, with the initiative's team members mobilized to focus on the most urgent health issue at hand. However, we should all be inspired by the example of how Professor Lewis and her colleagues remained committed, stayed the course and picked it up when things had normalized.

In closing, some argue that the implementation of value-based healthcare is progressing slowly and that the changes needed may be too challenging to be rolled out globally or even nationally. Transformational change can either be fast and disruptive or gradual, taking place over a longer period of time. Healthcare systems are inherently risk averse, avoiding disruption if possible. However, patients increasingly notice and resent this. There are a rapidly growing number of examples of value-based healthcare being successfully implemented across the globe, and Wales is one of the first places in which this is national and system-wide. From Professor Lewis's book it is clear that the programme has launched successfully and that roll-out has progressed well, but also that there is still a long way to go.

Most of the examples around the world have been led by passionate, fearless and purpose-driven individuals. Lewis is one such outstanding leader. But no matter how impressive you will find her story and how unwavering she has been in her push to improve the system for patients, none of you reading the book should step to the side, feeling that you 'could never have done that'. I believe that the author will convince you that it can be done – that we can learn from her and others to avoid some of their mistakes. We can do our part; we can take one step at a time. Wonderful quotes open each of the book's chapters, with one from Ursula K. Le Guin perfectly illustrating this point: 'You cannot buy the revolution. You cannot make the revolution. You can only be the revolution. It is in your spirit or it is nowhere.'

Finally, for readers in a healthcare leadership position, you should ask yourself how you can make it easier for Professor Lewis's kindred spirits to step forward. How can you do what her leaders did: encourage, equip, provide the resources and freedom to experiment, fail and drive improvement? Be bold and make it happen. We owe it to our grandchildren!

Dr Stefan Larsson, MD, PhD and new grandfather
Västerö, Sweden

Moral injury: why we must tackle the global crisis in healthcare

In 2012, on a typically busy Friday, I was sitting in my consulting room in my primary care practice in an old mining town in the South Wales valleys. I was on call, meaning that I could expect around sixty patient contacts between 8 a.m. and 6.30 p.m., forty-five of which would be face to face. I also had two scheduled house calls: one to an elderly man with complex comorbidities and no family living nearby; the other to a lady with cancer in the terminal phase of her illness. The latter was a lady who was very well known to me; she needed coordinated palliative care so that we could care for her at home in her dying days, as was her wish. I was stressed. There were a lot of problems to sort out and not enough time to handle them in the manner I would have wished.

Towards the end of the morning another of my regular patients came to see me. Janice was in her mid-fifties and had recently been diagnosed with a chronic pain syndrome. These debilitating conditions last for years and sometimes for life, often with a devastating impact on the quality of life of the sufferer. Traditional pain-relieving medications no longer work well and there are often other symptoms – mood and sleep disturbance, for example, or chronic fatigue – as well. Patients need a lot of support to help them manage their condition. Janice was not doing well. I wanted her to be able to access additional therapy and coaching to help her cope but the only available service to which Janice could be referred was 15 miles away.

Janice declined the referral. She was too debilitated to manage the two bus journeys that would get her there, and she could not afford a taxi. She was also highly sceptical that it would help (and, in truth, this was the main problem that I could not overcome), so she asked me to increase her pain medication. I was under pressure to get to my house calls and there was insufficient time to support Janice further. I was not meeting her needs and that did not feel good. I felt I had failed as a doctor and I experienced something I can only describe as an ache in my chest. Much later, I saw this uncomfortable and distressing feeling defined as 'moral injury'. The resources at my disposal were insufficient for delivering the standard of care I wished to give my patients.

As well as being the senior partner in my practice, I was also a Primary Care Clinical Director in my local integrated health board at that time. In that role I was involved in medicines optimization strategies and service transformation at a system level. About a week after seeing Janice I found myself in a board meeting in which there was intense scrutiny of prescribing variation in relation to chronic pain medication, specifically pregabalin. The drug was expensive at the time and it also had the potential to have harmful side effects if it was used incorrectly. The board – not unreasonably – wanted to take action to ensure prescribing was within guidelines, and I was alarmed to see that my practice was in the top five highest prescribers of pregabalin in the borough.

I thought about Janice and the high burden of disease in the community that my practice served – an area with a high level of socioeconomic deprivation. I began to feel intense frustration that we were using resources so ineffectively across a pathway of care and that we were not looking at this problem from the perspective of the patient and the outcomes that mattered. Often, we had little more than a prescription pad to help, and this fell far short of what was really needed to improve outcomes. For Janice, increasing the availability of non-pharmacological support for her condition could have improved her quality of life. It would have enabled me to reduce both her medication burden and the number of clinic visits with me, which had not helped her at all. It might even have helped her go back to work, or at least improved her social functioning and wellbeing. But we did not know that because we were not measuring outcomes.

Janice's needs were not being met, and nor were those of many others – and this was costing the system a great deal. Surely, we could do this better and improve outcomes, reduce costs and release healthcare professional capacity if only we took a whole-pathway perspective? Without realizing it, I was thinking about value-based healthcare. Value-based healthcare is a model of healthcare that focuses on improving the outcomes that matter to patients while managing system resources effectively. The more I thought about the issue, the more examples I could think of where outcomes could be vastly improved through relatively small changes to the way care was delivered. I became ever more frustrated.

*

Modern healthcare is entering a global crisis. We are spending more and more and yet the outcomes for people receiving care are not improving at a similar rate. In many places, the experience of care is also suffering, and inequities of access to care are a threat. Healthcare professionals are increasingly beleaguered and many want to quit, yet our populations are predicted to need ever-increasing numbers of them if we are to meet the changing health needs of societies everywhere. Meanwhile, the affordability of exciting new medical technologies, such as cell and gene therapies, is in doubt.

Through its focus on outcomes that matter, and the relative costs of achieving those outcomes across whole pathways of care, value-based care has become an attractive approach to tackling some of these 'wicked problems'. Radical changes to the way we deliver care are needed if we are to sustainably and equitably support people who are living for many years with chronic disease and if we are to be able to afford innovative new technologies in medicine.

Change is hard. There is no panacea for addressing the complexity of the problems that healthcare faces. However, the principles of value-based healthcare – a focus on what matters to patients along with data-driven decision making – are the best approach we have. It has become a beacon of hope to those principled individuals striving to make healthcare work for patients and for those creating health policy for the future.

This book is a how-to manual for every practitioner and healthcare service provider who wants to improve both outcomes for patients and the sustainability of our healthcare systems, wherever they may reside. It is for anyone who, like me, has found themselves frustrated by the roadblocks that are preventing them from achieving those goals. It is also a very personal story that draws on the many lessons learned in the Welsh health service, where value-based healthcare was first embarked upon ten years ago. These lessons are applicable around the globe.

This guide to implementing value-based healthcare is written in three parts.

Part I (chapters 1–3) tells the story of a small team attempting to implement value-based healthcare, first in a healthcare provider organization and then nationally (in Wales). It details the profound cultural and organizational changes that must take place in healthcare if value is to be achieved. The team implemented value-based healthcare through a process of experimentation, learning on the ground how best to engage colleagues and how to measure outcomes in practice. Finally, they learned how to embed value-based healthcare as central to the ethos of the healthcare system for the longer term and how to increase value for patients, providers and payers.

Part II (chapters 4–6) puts the learning into practice on the ground. Chapter 4 introduces a conceptual framework for looking at how we increase value at three levels: people, pathways of care, and populations. It continues by examining the essential incorporation of person-centred approaches to care if we are to achieve the outcomes that matter to us as individual people. Chapter 5 explains the myriad ways in which healthcare systems can drive value across whole pathways of care, including all the component parts for improving outcomes and managing precious system resources, financial or otherwise. Chapters 6 takes us up another level again, exploring value-based healthcare delivery for our populations. These chapters are brought to life by anecdotes and exemplars, drawing inspiration from learning in other contexts around the world to demonstrate that the principles of value-based healthcare can be applied anywhere.

Part III delves into both the organizational prerequisites and the infrastructure that are needed to make value-based healthcare possible. Value-based healthcare is a data-driven discipline, and chapter 7 is therefore dedicated to addressing the challenges of collecting, combining, analysing, visualizing and using data to make better decisions. The book's final chapter reflects on some of the pitfalls encountered when implementing value-based healthcare, and it looks at what needs to happen now if we are to achieve better outcomes for all and sustainable healthcare into the future.

One of the most powerful lessons from the implementation of value-based healthcare is the critical role played by multi-professional collaboration. Throughout this book you will find vignettes describing the background, role and personal motivations of some of the main protagonists in taking forward the mammoth task of implementation. Without the kind of commitment and collaborative leadership that they have provided, it is almost impossible to overcome the cultural, technical and practical barriers that present themselves as obstacles to value-based healthcare.

Acknowledgements

There are a great many people who have made the creation of this book possible. First, the extraordinary group of individuals who have been with me on the value-based healthcare journey since 2013. Some of them are mentioned in the book, but there are many. I would like to begin by thanking the protagonists in the book who agreed to be interviewed. I believe their testimonies bring the text to life. Thank you to Alan, Adele, Hamish, Allan, Helen and Imran.

The early work of value-based healthcare in the Aneurin Bevan Health Board was rooted in primary care. From that era, I would like to thank Alan Brace, Paul Buss, Adele Cahill and the value-based healthcare team; and Liam Taylor and the rest of our primary care team: Kartik Hariharan, Gareth Roberts, David Minton, Rob Holcombe and Caroline Mills. My experiences as a GP in the South Wales Valleys shaped the value-based healthcare work in Wales, especially my life at Glan Rhyd surgery. I would like to thank my colleagues there, and my patients, from whom I learned many hard lessons about healthcare.

ICHOM have been a constant presence throughout, starting with their early support for the implementation of outcomes measurement. Nowadays, my relationship with ICHOM is a true partnership, driven as we are by the same mission of improving outcomes for patients and value for healthcare systems. I would particularly like to thank Christina Akkerman, Thomas Kelley and Jennifer Bright, along with all the team past and present.

The Welsh Value in Health Centre and the wider team embedded within CEDAR and Digital Health and Care Wales may be small in number but they are huge in heart and skill, and they have overcome seemingly insurmountable barriers to build the infrastructure for value-based healthcare in Wales. I express my sincere gratitude to all members of the team. Ultimately, the success or failure of value-based healthcare rests with clinical operational teams in healthcare provider organizations. I thank the value-based healthcare teams in each of the health boards, and all the clinical teams and executive boards involved in this work. There was limited space in the book for describing their exceptional work and I know there is so much more that could have been included.

This is my first book and I am grateful for the support that has been given to me throughout from friends and colleagues, especially Mike and Marie Mount, Jennifer Burgos, Sophie Clarke, Antonio Weiss, Sarah Busby, Sharath Jeevan, Joseph Casey, Lucy Pocock, Peter Weeks and Meinir Jones. Thank you to all those who have provided images and case studies for the book: Sarah Puntoni, Said Shadi, Sally Cox and her team at Digital Health and Care Wales, Chris Lambert, Mel Thomas, Claire Dunstan, Kerith Jones and Pieter de Bey. I also owe immense gratitude to Stefan Larsson for writing the foreword: his generosity, mentorship and attention to detail has added a great deal to the book.

I could not believe my good fortune when London Publishing Partnership agreed to publish the book as part of their *Perspectives* series. Thank you to Sam Clark, Richard Baggaley and Diane Coyle for making the whole process so enjoyable.

My final tribute is to the growing network of people around the world who are working on value-based healthcare and related disciplines. They continue to provide inspiration and encouragement to me every day. Thank you.

PART I

A STORY OF VALUE-BASED HEALTHCARE IN PRACTICE

CHAPTER 1

Beginnings: the roots of value-based healthcare in Wales and beyond

'Always design a thing by considering it in its next larger context – a chair in a room, a room in a house, a house in an environment, an environment in a city plan.'
— Eliel Saarinen

Value-based healthcare is, in essence, a vehicle for transformational change in healthcare. Its principles, which are both very simple and universally valid, are that we should focus on improving the outcomes that matter to people and that we should eliminate unnecessary use of resources in healthcare systems. The application of these principles in different countries around the world depends a great deal on local context. This chapter sets the scene in Wales. It tells the story of how and why value-based healthcare became an important delivery mechanism for the nation's attempts to improve patient outcomes and tackle growing unsustainability in its healthcare system.

Healthcare is funded and delivered in different ways in different countries, and each population has diversity of culture, geography, language and need. Therefore, in applying these simple principles to diverse systems of healthcare around the world we cannot impose a single blueprint for change if we are to succeed in delivering value for our populations. Context is everything if we are to succeed in applying value-based principles in every setting: a clinician with a patient; that therapeutic consultation within a service; that service within an organization; that organization within a country's health ecosystem. In 2014, at the very beginning of value-based care in Wales, that context was a system that was increasingly struggling to cope with the rising health needs of an older and sicker population.

The Welsh context: prudent healthcare

In January 2014 the Minister for Health and Social Care in Wales, Professor Mark Drakeford, did something extraordinary, in political terms, when he announced the advent of prudent healthcare in Wales as a response to the emerging healthcare crisis.[1] It was, arguably, the first time a politician had publicly hinted that if we were both to achieve the outcomes that mattered to people and to support a sustainable system, we needed a different approach to modern healthcare delivery. The announcement paved the way for the later introduction of value-based healthcare in Wales, and it created fertile ground for its implementation.

The sentiment behind prudent healthcare was to work in partnership with patients and the public, encouraging their greater involvement in their health and care; to make best use of all available resources; to reduce waste; and to tackle unwarranted variation in care delivery (both overtreatment and undertreatment). This was the flagship policy of Professor Drakeford's first tenure as health minister and its development was supported by the Bevan Commission, a government-funded think tank in Wales.

As I was later to realize, the health policy context in Wales was already inherently helpful to the introduction of value-based healthcare because of the strategy set in the Well-being of Future Generations (Wales) Act 2015[2] and, later, in 'A healthier Wales',[3] the long-term strategy for health and social care in Wales. Both policies spoke of the need to focus on better outcomes and they came immediately before the move to national adoption of value-based healthcare in Wales. The Institute for Healthcare Improvement had been a significant influence on the Bevan Commission and on Welsh health policy for some time, so the 'Quadruple Aim' set out in 'A healthier Wales' – with its four targets of enhancing patient experience, improving population health, reducing costs and improving healthcare professional wellbeing – was often cited.[4]

After consultation, the Bevan Commission arrived at four principles of prudent healthcare that were intended to be a philosophy, or golden seam, running through health and social care policy, planning and resource allocation, and the delivery of healthcare services from the boardroom to the bedside. The overall ethos and the four principles were regarded as the driving forces behind a social movement by the architects of prudent healthcare.

The prudent healthcare principles are listed below.

1. Public and professionals are equal partners through coproduction.

2. Care for those with the greatest health need first.

3. Do only what is needed and do no harm.

4. Reduce inappropriate variation though evidence-based approaches.

There was broad support for the principles across the NHS in Wales and plans were drawn up for their adoption into practice. As a direct result of this I was appointed as Assistant Medical

Director for Prudent and Value-Based Healthcare by Dr Paul Buss and Alan Brace, the medical director and the director of finance of the Aneurin Bevan University Health Board, and I joined the Guiding Coalition for Prudent Healthcare in Welsh Government led by Dame Ruth Hussey, then the chief medical officer for Wales.

I started to think deeply about what prudent healthcare really meant to me, both as a practising GP and as the Assistant Medical Director involved with 'whole pathway' service transformation. For the first time, I began to observe how a well-considered policy initiative such as this plays out on the ground, and I could see that there was a problem with its implementation because of a lack of measurement. The system was not talking about measuring outcomes in 2014, despite describing them in its policy documents. Prudent healthcare was a movement – an underpinning philosophy – that was intended to improve patient outcomes and make better use of all resources in the Welsh NHS. But to know that those goals were being met, we needed value-based healthcare as an operational delivery mechanism.

Emerging movements around the world

Looking further afield, I could see that Wales was not alone in the problems it was facing. Professional movements had been springing up around the world for several years with the aim of tackling overlapping issues in healthcare such as waste, low-value care (care that does not contribute to a better patient outcome) and overmedicalization.

These movements tap into the notion that, for all our evidence-based pathways and guidelines, we regularly miss the point for the patient. This is often due to having insufficient time with the patient and therefore not being able to elicit their goals, preferences and needs for holistic care. We are in danger of becoming mechanistic and formulaic in our approach to evidence-based healthcare, relying too much on algorithms with the inevitable consequence of overconsumption and waste without improved outcomes. The trick is to strike the right balance between evidence-based standardization of processes of healthcare and person-centred care – a goal that is, of course, true to David Sackett's full definition of evidence-base medicine in the 1990s.[5] We will come back to this tension in more detail in a later chapter, but in essence it is only by capturing and understanding clinical and patient-reported outcomes that we can make a judgment about whether we are getting care right.

First, let us explore some of the other relevant global movements.

Slow medicine – founded in Italy and born out of the slow food movement – emphasizes 'measured, respectable and equitable' care. It focuses on a person-centred approach, with sufficient time given to the holistic needs of the patient. It has the dual aim of improving outcomes and reducing unnecessary and potentially harmful overmedicalization.[6]

Choosing Wisely International[7] was created by the American Board of Internal Medicine in 2012 to curtail the growth in unnecessary diagnostic tests and treatments in the United States, and it now has a broad network of physician exponents around the world. Dr Jessica Otte, an inspirational family physician from Canada, has brought elements of the choosing wisely and slow medicine concepts together into 'Less is More Medicine'. Soon after prudent healthcare was launched in Wales, Realistic Medicine – a major policy initiative with a very similar perspective – was championed by the office of the chief medical officer in Scotland.[8]

We can start to see some key recurring themes in all of this: the need for person-centred care; for reducing unwarranted variation in care processes (often through quality improvement methodologies); and for reducing waste and harm. As we shall see throughout this book, each of these themes represents an important component of the quest to increase value in healthcare for patients, professionals and the wider healthcare system. These professional movements are important because they represent disquiet within a medical profession that knows it can do better for its patients. These are early signs of the necessary cultural shift to implementing value-based healthcare.

The Getting It Right First Time (GIRFT) programme[9] is a wide-ranging programme of work developed by NHS England and championed by the orthopaedic surgeon Professor Tim Briggs. It is a clinically led and data-driven approach to reducing unwarranted variation in care processes, many of which are strongly linked to patient safety and outcomes as well as costs in healthcare delivery. It is of great importance here because, while it is a programme of work rather than a movement like the others mentioned, it introduces two new elements that are critical to the delivery of value-based healthcare: clinical leadership through networks; and data-driven approaches to decision making. The latter enable the development of learning health and care systems, which we will discuss later in the book.

I began to think in depth about how to take the concepts born out of these movements and apply them to the day-to-day business of healthcare delivery across the continuum of care, from the community to the hospital and back again. This started with an analysis of our own prudent healthcare concepts.

Putting the four principles into practice

Principle 1. Public and professionals are equal partners through coproduction

Coproduction, like any word that is adopted into policy or management processes, can often feel like a rather hackneyed term and is not universally popular. However, the concept it describes is extremely important to the delivery of modern healthcare services and for improving the experience and outcomes of the people using those services. Here is a definition of coproduction from the UK's Social Care Institute for Excellence:

A way of working whereby citizens and decision makers, or people who use services, family carers and service providers work together to create a decision or service which works for them all.

For this principle to be applied in the context of prudent healthcare we must consider to what extent people are (and feel) involved in caring for their health. This can be viewed as an individual's participation in their care (the micro level) and as public/patient involvement in service design (the macro level).

At a micro level, coproduction refers to shared decision making.[10] This is the process by which healthcare professionals help people make choices about their health and care. Doing this well requires time; it often takes in multiple consultations; and ideally it utilizes the differing skill sets of a multidisciplinary team. The process should include discussions not only about therapeutic interventions, such as prescribing medicines or surgery, but also about when/if to have a scan or take a holiday or undertake any other activity that is important to that person. All trade-offs in that decision-making process should be explored and understood. It is all too easy to fall into the trap of jumping to conclusions about what our patients' priorities are and what really matters, perhaps focusing solely on the clinical outcomes as seen through the eyes of the clinician.

There are several necessary steps in the shared decision-making process.

- There needs to be a realistic shared view of the situation. One that considers cues from the individual on the amount of information that is shared and the pace at which that sharing is done, and takes into account the degree of self-efficacy and health literacy.

- An appreciation of psychosocial and other contextual factors is required. For example, the person's family and work circumstances should be considered. Do they have a support network?

- The patient's fears, beliefs, expectations, wants, needs and goals should be explored. For example, are we on the same page regarding the diagnosis, the potential prognosis and what matters most to the person receiving care? Only then can we support a person to achieve what is important to them.

- Shared goal setting is required.

- It is necessary to impart understanding of the treatment options and choices available and to acknowledge uncertainty. We do not always know what the outcome of a decision will be, and we need to make patients aware of that and also explain the risks associated with each course of action.

As clinicians we must continuously check our self-awareness because we tend to default to 'doing something' – often with the best of intentions – before understanding whether that is what the person we are treating would choose or whether it is in their best interests. Taking this step back can be difficult as we want the best outcomes for those we care for, and we do not like to fail. We are often afraid of censure if our decision making is later judged to be wrong, and this sometimes leads us to over test and over treat. We often have too little time to meet the holistic needs of the person sitting before us. Good coproduction is therefore most likely to occur when the multidisciplinary team work together seamlessly across the whole system to support the individual throughout their treatment and beyond. As the number of us with multiple comorbidities grows, the importance of an expert generalist becomes even more important in guiding individuals to make the best possible decisions in their own context. As Atul Gawande says in his book *Being Mortal*: 'Life is choices. They are relentless.'[11]

At a macro level, the public must be given the opportunity to make a direct contribution to the design of local services so that they are meaningful to them and meet their needs. It is fair to say that we have a long way to go before we achieve this to a high standard in all areas. In promoting public health and sustaining our healthcare system we should seek to reach a balance between the rights and responsibilities of individuals. This brings into question the experience of public services and the fostering of a sense of community, but there is also an onus on service providers to promote equality, diversity, accessibility and reciprocity when embarking on the coproductive process. When these pillars are not in place, the process is tokenistic; it is of limited value; and it tends, entirely understandably, to disengage those involved.

When done well, coproduction begins with active listening, and the subsequent interaction between the involved groups produces a rich seam of information that can inform a much-improved patient experience and better, more innovative and flexible ways of meeting the healthcare needs of the population in question.

If we adopt the approach detailed above in its entirety, we will surely have a better chance of improving patient experience and healthcare outcomes, and we will go some way towards creating a sustainable health service for the future. Surely, then, coproduction is something we must take very seriously indeed.

Principle 2. Care for those with the greatest health need first

At first glance, principle 2 seems obvious and straightforward to adopt. After all, who would deny that we should prioritize those in greatest need of care? As we consider this more carefully, however, we start to see that this is not at all as easy as it first appears. Do we really focus our resources and attention on those with greatest need? How do we define need?

When treatment is immediately lifesaving, we can reassure ourselves that we are certainly prioritizing those in greatest need, and the United Kingdom's National Health Service excels in this function, but what about when the situation is less of an emergency? For example, in a healthcare system where resources will always be finite, how do we prioritize. We must use the best available evidence in our decision making, always considering the opportunity cost and the impact on other people. Doing this means we need to measure the health outcomes we are achieving with our patients, not just the degree to which patients can access services.

This principle also steers us towards promoting equity in health and reducing health inequalities. Equity is defined as 'the absence of avoidable or remediable differences among groups of people, whether those groups are defined socially, economically, demographically or geographically'.[12] Equity has us striving to achieve equal outcomes. It is distinct from equality, which implies that everyone has access to the same resources. Those in greater need may require more than those who are in a privileged position if they are to achieve the same outcome. If we are to achieve equity, a greater focus on certain demographic groups is needed to achieve better health, and this goes beyond healthcare itself, encompassing housing, education and other needs. It also requires a separate approach for those living with rare diseases.[13]

Aristotle himself described the need for disproportionate provision in favour of those with greater need in his theory of distributive justice, and yet the 'inverse care law' still exists now, despite our best efforts to reverse it. The inverse care law was first proposed by Dr Julian Tudor-Hart in 1971 based on research into the population of his general practice in the South Wales valleys.[14] It states that the availability of good medical or social care tends to vary inversely with the needs of the population served. As a South Wales GP myself, this resonates more than it should half a century later. Health inequalities in the South Wales valleys have not lessened during my lifetime.

We would do well to remember that those in greatest need often have the quietest voice. In healthcare we must therefore be strong advocates for the vulnerable if we are to reduce health inequalities.

Healthcare systems are full of targets. These are well intentioned and designed to get the best possible performance out of systems. They often relate to important time-based metrics such as the length of time patients spend waiting for appointments or the length of hospital stays. We must guard against unintended perverse consequences, though, as, paradoxically, some targets can cause us to have the wrong focus and steer us away from a focus on improving outcomes. In other words, what gets measured gets done. And if we fail to measure outcomes and use outcome data, we will not be focused on improving those outcomes.

Finally, there is always the deeply personal and emotive tension between individual and population need. When I am sitting in my surgery with a person in my care, I am thinking about their needs and how I can help address them. I am not necessarily thinking about the whole population of my GP practice, any more than I would if a member of my own family was ill. This is the power of human interaction and advocacy, and we would never want to sacrifice that. And yet, we all have a responsibility for the wider population.

In a national context, we must consider that an expensive new intervention with marginal benefit could displace invisible activity that benefits other individuals. Unfortunately, cost effectiveness is not equivalent to affordability, and the latter is not within the remit of health technology assessment organizations to comment upon. Something and somebody always suffer because of this displacement, and this issue is only set to worsen as we sail further into the perfect storm that healthcare faces. In the book *The Patient Priority*,[15] this storm is described as crises in healthcare that relate to value, evidence and purpose. There are seminal points to take away from this analysis. The increasing spend in healthcare (including growth in biomedical research) is not linked to a similar gain in patient outcomes, and it is becoming unaffordable and unsustainable everywhere. Increasing biomedical knowledge has led to more and more guidelines, not all of which are conclusively linked to improved outcomes. Patients and clinicians are struggling in the resultant complex and malfunctioning systems. None of this is easy.

I have concluded that this is the most challenging prudent healthcare principle of all, and it is one that healthcare professionals cannot solve alone. What matters most in healthcare and how will we afford it? We need honesty, and there needs to be a debate that includes politicians, journalists, professionals and the public if we are to sustain our system. As I had discovered, Wales was not alone in experiencing these challenges in healthcare. Colleagues from all over the world were describing issues relating to poor outcomes, unsustainability and workforce burnout – these problems just manifested themselves slightly differently depending on the national context.

Principle 3. Do only what is needed and do no harm

I have a feeling that the illustrious French philosopher Voltaire was not particularly impressed with doctors when he gave us the following two pearls of wisdom:

- 'doctors pour drugs of which they know little to cure disease of which they know less, into humans of whom they know nothing'; and

- 'the art of medicine consists in amusing the patient whilst nature cures the disease'.

Perhaps he had been on the receiving end of an adverse effect of a preferred remedy of the day, or maybe he had been attacked by a quack bearing a jar of leeches. I don't know. However, I do think he was making a point that still holds true today, even with the advances we have made in our knowledge and understanding of disease and with the development of evidence-based modern medicine. The uncomfortable truth is that modern healthcare still has, at best, a propensity for overselling some of its benefits and, at worst, for actually causing harm.

When the prudent healthcare principles were first described, some of my colleagues felt a little wounded at what principle 3 was implying. 'Of course we don't intentionally do harm' was one common response. 'Are you suggesting we do things that aren't needed?' and 'We follow guidelines and pathways after all' were too. This hurts us as physicians because it goes straight to the core of our values. All of us want to help – to make things better for those we care for – and we have a lot of guidelines to help us to do that. But in all this there is a danger that we as clinicians default to a guideline intervention before fully knowing the human being in front of us: we need to understand their needs, their goals and their aspirations, and we have to be clear about whether that intervention will create the desired outcome.

What is wrong with that, I hear you ask. We are following the guidelines. The problem is that there is a risk–benefit equation underlying all healthcare that we deliver to our patients. There are inherent problems with applying single-disease guidelines to people with complex needs, particularly where the evidence quality is low. There is always a risk of harm when we intervene, so surely we need to truly ascertain our patients' health goals and look for the least invasive way of achieving them? In so doing we are bound to reduce harm and improve outcomes while still practising evidence-based medicine. The goals and the solutions needed to reach those goals must be arrived at together having considered the best available evidence.

Harm caused by healthcare (iatrogenic harm) is both visible and invisible. Serious drug reactions, hospital-acquired infections, surgical complications and medical errors are easier to identify. Less so the effects of polypharmacy (too many drugs), of over testing and imaging, or of pursuing treatment that may prove a greater burden than the disease. Iatrogenesis is from the

Greek meaning 'brought forth by the healer'. Let us bring forth as little harm as possible and prove that rascal Voltaire wrong.

Principle 4. Reduce inappropriate variation through evidence-based approaches

The way in which we receive language can be very personal, and as the prudent healthcare story unfolded it was interesting to observe the power that words have, both to please and to offend. I confess that I was offended by the word 'inappropriate' as it appears in the fourth prudent principle. I have thought about why that was and have concluded that 'inappropriate' somehow implies a transgression – in this case perhaps by a well-meaning healthcare professional. That was my interpretation at least, and I believe 'unwarranted' would be better and is, in any case, truer to the original definition.

This may seem like a trivial point but it became important much later when trying to engage healthcare professionals in value-based healthcare approaches and to explain these principles to them in a way that resonated with their values. Unwarranted variation is a term coined by Dr John Wennberg, founder of the Centre for Evaluative Clinical Services at Dartmouth Medical School in the United States. He defined it as 'variation in healthcare delivery that cannot be explained by illness, medical need or evidence'.

The idea that we should identify and reduce variation in healthcare is decades old and has been worked on by many well-known figures in modern healthcare.[16] So what is variation, why should we tackle it and what does doing so mean for clinicians and the people they care for? There are several different types of variation – some warranted and some not. This is an important consideration when we analyse variation data (processes, outcomes and costs), when we think about the causes of the variation we are seeing, and when we decide how to act upon it. Let us look at three examples in detail.

(1) Effective care
Here we are talking about situations in which approaches that are known to be safe and effective, i.e. where there is a strong link to better outcomes for patients, are not used. Examples of this include

- variation in patients with atrial fibrillation receiving anticoagulation to prevent stroke;

- variation in adherence to surgical checklists to reduce errors and improve safety in theatre; and

- underuse of retinopathy screening for people with diabetes to prevent sight loss.

Variation of this type may require quality improvement measures to improve clinical care or an investment in services by the healthcare organization. This is a type of unwarranted variation. We can clearly see that improving outcomes, and therefore value, is everybody's business. Understanding the cause of the variation is critical to deploying the correct solution.

(2) Preference-sensitive care
This refers to types of care where there are often trade-offs between the benefits and risks of the intervention. Consequently, the quality of shared decision making must be high if the best outcomes are to achieved, with the individual being aided by their clinician in navigating the current evidence base and arriving at the best choice for their context. Examples could be knee replacement surgery or treatment choices in early prostate cancer. The aim here is to remove as much clinician bias as possible, and this can lead to warranted variation in care that is based on patient preference and choice. The patient should ask themselves, 'For somebody like me, am I more likely to achieve the outcome I want with or without surgery for my knee

arthritis?' Or, in the case of early prostate cancer, where watchful waiting and monitoring is an option to be considered alongside more aggressive treatment, 'How do I feel about that?'

(3) Supply-sensitive care

Supply-sensitive care tends to be professionally or system driven care and it can result in an overuse of healthcare that is not beneficial to patients. A good example of this is seen in outpatient follow-up appointments where, historically, the system has a tendency to sequentially follow people up at arbitrary intervals irrespective of whether they are currently well or in urgent need. Sometimes this also refers to the ongoing practice of an intervention that new evidence has now shown to be less effective than previously thought. Evidence-based medicine is defined as 'the conscientious, explicit, and judicious use of current best evidence in making decisions about the care of individual patients'.[17] We know that medical practice is notoriously slow to adapt to new knowledge, particularly in abandoning outmoded interventions that have now been found to be of limited benefit.

*

The reasons why we need to tackle unwarranted variation should now be clear: it can lead to harm and it leads to waste and higher costs, so we must do our best to reduce it if we are to create a sustainable healthcare system. This is why it is discussed in prudent healthcare, Realistic Medicine and other similar initiatives. But we need to be careful. Our information is often incomplete and, in some areas, variation data often raises more questions than it immediately answers. When we are looking at referral and prescribing data from primary care, for example, there may be external reasons for variation, such as a lack of alternatives on offer. This has certainly been the case in mental health, where we have seen huge growth in antidepressant prescribing linked to the lack of availability of talking therapies. We simply do not yet have the means to reliably capture variation due to patient preference, or to understand to what extent clinician behaviour is influenced by requests from patients to refer, test or prescribe. We need to better understand real-world patient outcomes and we must seek to reduce unwarranted variation in those outcomes, making sure that we are making true comparisons.

We still need to tackle unwarranted variation, but we need to do so sensitively and with great care. Most of all we must look at the system through the eyes of a person needing care. The only way we will truly understand if variation is good or bad is by measuring the outcomes that result from the care we are giving our patients. Supporting people to make good choices to meet their health goals and giving them the ability to lead their own care and maintain as much independence as possible will help us deliver the right care at the right time and achieve the best possible outcomes in partnership with our patients.

Overcoming obstacles on the ground: prudent healthcare's many challenges

Given the degree to which all participants – patient groups, healthcare professionals, managers and policymakers – bought into prudent healthcare, it would be tempting to think that putting it into practice would be easy. However, each of the principles requires a radical shift in the way things are done in healthcare – a shift that requires concerted effort, collaboration and resourcing across the system.

Within the health boards, prudent healthcare was often described as a separate workstream rather than a golden seam running through every plan and service transformation. Worse, cost improvement targets that were put against the interventions described were both highly unrealistic and not triangulated with outcome data. Prudent healthcare does save money (as well as workforce time and other resources) but we cannot say it is succeeding unless we improve, or at least maintain, outcomes.

Another significant and common problem with the way prudent healthcare was implemented was that it was usually tackled as solely a service problem rather than a system problem. That is, there was no attempt to look at the whole pathway or continuum of care. This meant that there were many missed opportunities to 'shift left'. Shifting left is a frequently used phrase in healthcare transformation that refers to two concepts: first, the ability to move care out of the hospital and closer to patients' homes in primary and community care; and second, moving from a reactive approach to healthcare, where people are 'rescued' in the hospital after a crisis or emergency, to a proactive approach to prevention, timely diagnosis and good chronic disease management, the latter seeking to mitigate against preventable exacerbations of disease.

Finally, there was too much focus on stewardship of resources by doctors rather than shared responsibility across the whole system for optimum resource use, reduction of waste and improvement in outcomes. And, of course, we did not really understand whether we were achieving the outcomes that mattered to our patients so how could we know if we were being prudent?

What we needed was both a delivery mechanism for prudent healthcare principles and a measurement system. That combination was value-based healthcare.

There were some in the system that viewed prudent healthcare simply as a way of tackling a perceived overconsumption of resources by the medical profession rather than as a better way of meeting the needs of patients. We should not pretend that overconsumption of resources (or waste) is not an issue. It is any intervention that uses up time or resource that was not needed to achieve the desired outcome for the patient, e.g. an unnecessary appointment, scan or treatment. Worse still, some unnecessary treatments result in a degree of harm to the patient: a side effect of an unnecessary treatment, for example. Overconsumption is therefore an important topic. But it should never be seen in isolation. Of equal importance are the positive actions we must take to meet patients' needs and improve outcomes.

One of the striking features of the organization I was working in at the time was the strong, emerging relationship between the medical director and the finance director, each seeking to understand each other's worlds so that better collective decisions could be made at the board level. I found myself reflecting on the importance of fostering multiprofessional collaboration if we are to improve outcomes and reduce costs in healthcare. It was fascinating to watch how the collaboration between the medical director Paul Buss and the chief financial officer Alan Brace was becoming such a powerful vehicle for change, with Alan often talking about patient outcomes and Paul frequently referencing costing and stewardship of resources. They were modelling how effective a partnership approach could be in addressing the wickedest of healthcare organizational problems.

I did not know it at the time, but this was a perfect illustration of one of the central tenets of Michael Porter and Elizabeth Teisberg's theory and a quote from their book *Redefining Health Care*: 'Value is the only goal that can unite the interests of all system participants.'[18] None of us as individuals, and no single profession, can achieve radical healthcare transformation alone. We must work it out together or we will fail apart.

The seeds of value-based healthcare

In parallel with the work on prudent healthcare, Alan had begun to talk to me about value-based healthcare and his time at Harvard learning about the work of Porter and Teisberg. He also introduced me to the newly formed International Consortium for Health Outcomes Measurement (ICHOM), pioneers in bringing together experts and patients on outcome measurement. I was appointed as the generalist physician on the ICHOM working group to define the standard set of outcomes for hip and knee arthritis.[19] This transcontinental work was carried out via telephone conference over a nine-month period. During the course of the project, the penny dropped for me. We had all these good intentions through the concepts of prudent healthcare and other movements, but we did not understand the outcomes that mattered. Neither did we use the right data to drive decision making in a true learning health and care system.

Structural arrangements in the Welsh NHS

At this point it is necessary to highlight the way that the National Health Service in Wales is structured and funded because this had a major bearing on how value-based principles were adopted into the system. We have since seen the evolution of similar approaches to value-based healthcare delivery across Europe and the Middle East, taking into account population health and the equitable attainment of outcomes that matter for every citizen. The context and culture of a country and healthcare system structure must be considered while taking a value-based approach to care, otherwise the approach is likely to meet insurmountable obstacles and founder in the early stages of the work.

Since 1999, all decision making in respect of healthcare delivery has been devolved from the UK government to the Welsh government, along with education, transport and local government, including social services. Healthcare is funded through public taxation and the Welsh government is the single payer, receiving a capitation-based allocation from Westminster based on the Barnett formula. The Barnett formula is an old and much-criticized mechanism for adjusting the Welsh block grant, and it is intended to reflect changes in public spending in England.

A helpful and interesting comparative analysis of the four UK health systems was undertaken by the OECD in 2016, looking at the impact of divergence in the structures.[5] Health consumes a growing proportion of the devolved budget allocation from the UK government in Westminster. In 2024/25 this equates to roughly £11.4 billion in revenue for Wales – over half the total allocated revenue for devolved services. There is a real danger that further rises in healthcare costs continue to erode funding for the very things that create health and prosperity, particularly education, transport and leisure. A more immediate problem is the negative impact on social care spending, which is funded through the local government share of the allocation. Inadequate social care provision places added pressures on the healthcare system because timely access to social care is necessary to support hospital discharges for those requiring residential care or additional support at home. Increasing urgency around tackling poor health outcomes, rising costs and health inequalities were therefore the major drivers for the development and adoption of prudent and value-based healthcare in Wales.

Through a further allocation formula, the Welsh health budget is allocated to the health organizations: seven integrated local health boards and three trusts (a specialist cancer centre, Public Health Wales and the Welsh ambulance service). Digital Health and Care Wales and Health Education and Improvement Wales are special health authorities overseeing digital and workforce development, respectively. Shared Services Partnership oversees the procurement activity of NHS Wales, and the Joint Commissioning Committee holds a budget with which it directly commissions highly specialized services on behalf of the integrated health boards. There is very little private healthcare in Wales.

Primary care has a ringfenced allocation and is largely delivered by independent contractors for whom the health boards manage the contracts. Despite the need to invest further in prevention and in keeping people with chronic illness well in the community, the proportion of spend from the overall budget going to this sector has not increased in real terms in decades. There is very little fee for service – in other words, healthcare professionals and providers are not paid for activity such as clinic visits or operations. They are instead expected to plan to meet the total needs of the population they are serving through the block allocation. There are very few incentives for high-quality care beyond a few remnants of the Quality and Outcomes Framework for general practice. Initiated throughout the United Kingdom in 2003/4, this scheme rewarded primary care practices on the achievement of certain quality indicators, including the attainment of clinical targets for chronic diseases such as hypertension and diabetes.

Participation in the work to define the standard set of outcomes for hip and knee arthritis piqued my curiosity about ICHOM, and I was keen to meet my fellow working group members and be there in person at Harvard Business School for the launch of their standard set of outcome measures. I therefore self-funded to attend the third ICHOM conference in Boston in 2014, allowing me to be there in person for the launch of the set at Harvard Business School. It was unbelievably energizing and it made a big impression on me. I returned to the United Kingdom convinced that a focus on outcomes, costs and a value-based approach to care was the obvious and natural delivery mechanism for prudent healthcare and the related movements with which I was becoming involved.

On my return, Alan called me into his office and asked me if I was up for a challenge. Would I go away with a blank sheet of paper and find out what it would take to make the Aneurin Bevan University Health Board an organization run on the principles of value-based healthcare? How could I refuse such an offer?

Alan Brace: driving a new paradigm

Much earlier in his career, Alan was already becoming an individual who challenged the paradigm of being a finance professional. He had an intense curiosity about the world of the clinician, and he spent a lot of time with clinical teams to gain an understanding of care delivery. His leadership was frequently boundary spanning and his roles often reached outside of his immediate financial brief into general management and even informatics. Pivotal to his later thinking were two periods: a spell working in West Wales with community services and talking to GPs; and some time spent in government. Interviewing Alan years later he says that through these experiences, he 'began to see the big picture'. He went on: 'Then in 1999 I had the opportunity to go to Harvard for three months to study on their general manager programme. Learning with such a diverse group of international professionals really broadened my thinking.'

By 2009 Alan was the director of finance for the newly formed Aneurin Bevan Health Board. The financial crash of the year before was beginning to impact on public services and Alan was focused on 'lean' methodology to create greater process efficiency and make cost improvements in the organization. He recalls becoming more and more weary of traditional approaches to cost reduction, feeling that they were increasingly ineffective. He also knew that they were not engaging to his clinical colleagues. He was drawn to a more strategic approach and found himself again reading the works of Michael Porter – this time his collaboration with Elizabeth Teisberg relating to value-based healthcare. In December 2013 he again found himself in Harvard, learning the principles of value-based care with a bunch of clinicians. He returned to Wales convinced that his organization needed to a focus on outcomes (both clinical and patient-reported) if it were to drive value and sustainability.

I asked Alan if he had a plan or a vision of what this would look like for us in the Aneurin Bevan Health Board and this was his response:

Initially I wanted to allow for organic growth of the idea and did not define an endpoint. I engaged early with significant executive and non-executive members of the board, notably Paul Buss the medical director and Andrew Goodall the CEO, and communicated progress to them regularly. I also had discussions with senior figures in Welsh government. I knew that I needed to form a small 'guiding coalition' of individuals who would just get on and do it. I knew we needed to measure outcomes and saw that we would benefit from ICHOM's help.

Thinking back, Alan also reflected on the importance of keeping a 'true north' and not veering off course if we want to effect change in healthcare. He saw his job as an enabler, moving obstacles out of the team's way, facilitating with resources where he could. He also protected us from considerable 'noise and criticism' within the organization in the early days. Key to this was enabling the value-based healthcare project to operate outside of standard operational governance until it grew legs. Up until that moment the team reported directly to the board. This was bottom-up work with very strong top-down support from the outset.

In 2017 Alan became director of finance for NHS Wales and for the Welsh government's Health and Social Services division, and he began to prepare the ground for value-based healthcare at a national scale.

Key lessons from chapter 1

Value-based healthcare focus

Value-based healthcare prioritizes outcomes that matter to patients at an individual level and at a population level. It seeks to help achieve balance in the inherent tension between these two aims. Equity is a core tenet, and resources should be allocated to address the needs of underserved populations so that everyone has the same opportunity to achieve the best healthcare outcome.

Multidisciplinary collaboration

Effective value-based healthcare implementation requires collaboration across all levels of the healthcare system, involving clinicians, finance professionals and policymakers to align resources with outcomes. It is not the sole preserve of any one professional group.

Strategic policy foundations

A supportive policy framework is critical for the long-term adoption of value-based healthcare in health systems internationally, and it must sit outside short-term political cycles.

Value-based healthcare implementation must consider the entire care pathway (from prevention through to palliative care) rather than isolated services or institutions. In this way, value-based healthcare supports integrated approaches to care.

Global movements

Movements born in different countries – Choosing Wisely, Slow Medicine and Realistic Medicine, for example – underline recurring themes of preventing disease, patient-centred care, reducing waste and prioritizing equity. Their goals are complementary to the value-based healthcare ethos, and there is strength in bringing supporters of these related approaches together under value-based healthcare.

CHAPTER 2

Velvet bulldozers: getting vaue-based healthcare off the ground

'He who has a strong enough why will find the how.'
— Viktor Frankl

Creating momentum towards value-based healthcare

Change is difficult, and nowhere is this more true than in a complex industry such as healthcare. From early on in our value-based healthcare journey, we benefited from the support and encouragement of influential people outside Wales. This helped us to retain momentum and confidence in pursuit of the innovative changes we wanted to make in the system. The president of the International Consortium for Health Outcomes Measurement (ICHOM), Dr Christina Akkerman, was one such person.

I remember sharing a taxi with Christina back in 2016 as we were travelling to a meeting together. She turned to me and said that we needed to be 'velvet bulldozers' in our pursuit of transformational change. This remark (and the soft stubbornness it engenders) has remained with me ever since. As we shall see throughout this book, there are many obstacles to transformational change. What is required is gentle but determined diplomacy and persistence in both moving those obstacles out of the way and bringing people along with the change.

Engaging the system with external 'superstars' had other benefits too. Outside big-name supporters can often create a level of excitement and confidence in a new system that is difficult to achieve from the inside, even if they are saying exactly the same things you are. Perhaps what they say about an expert simply being 'somebody from out of town with slides' is really true!

This chapter describes the lessons learned from the early days of value-based healthcare implementation, including the development of those early strategic partnerships.

Creating a search team: a period of learning

Shortly after asking me to lead the work on value-based healthcare, Alan announced two exciting developments. First, we would be forming a strategic partnership with the ICHOM,[1] engaging its support in helping us test the feasibility of measuring patient-reported outcomes in the Aneurin Bevan Health Board. And second, I was to be sent to Harvard Business School to attend the Executive Education Short Course on value-based healthcare. It is hard to express the sense of responsibility and privilege I felt.

Alan then made one more key move when he introduced me to Adele Cahill, an experienced procurement professional and manager with significant experience of managing change. Adele and I were to work together and take forward the value-based healthcare agenda. Alan did not specify what that would mean (I don't think any of us knew at that point what it would entail exactly), but he trusted us to do the right things. This early freedom to act was a critical factor in the subsequent momentum for value-based healthcare in Wales because it gave us license to be agile in our approach. We were also able to bypass some of the clunky bureaucracy always seen in large organizations, enabling us to make rapid progress with the work, particularly with securing the necessary resources to begin measuring outcomes.

Adele Cahill: putting the system under the microscope

Before entering the world of value-based healthcare, Adele Cahill had 30 years of experience as a procurement professional in NHS Wales under her belt. She was at the top of her game, having attained the position of deputy director in NHSWSSP, the organization that coordinated national procurements for the NHS in Wales. Reflecting now, she can see that she had always focused on price reduction when procuring goods and services, getting the best deal for patients but with little thought to the patient outcomes achieved. She was very effective at this too; she was considered a fearsome negotiator.

After many years in the trade, though, she had begun to develop a sense of unease that the continuous chasing of the pound or dollar was not making the difference she wanted to see in the system. Ultimately, she had begun to find it all a bit soul destroying. Something then happened to Adele that would solidify her view that we needed to think about procuring care differently.

Adele's mother became sick after a routine hospital procedure, and she was found to have severe *Clostridium difficile*, a hospital-acquired infection. She had uncontrollable diarrhoea forty to fifty times per day, so careful and attentive nursing was vital. To manage the situation, the nursing team were using incontinence pads, but the ones that were available were not sufficient to manage the large amounts of fluid and six or seven of them therefore had to be taped together.

Adele thought this was odd and went to the product catalogue to see if there was a better solution for her mother and indeed there was. It was possible to procure much larger continence sheets that would have had greater absorbency and provided more comfort. She went to the nursing team and suggested it. They replied that they were not allowed to order the product Adele had found because it was too expensive. It was clear that nobody had factored in patient outcome, product volumes used or nursing staff time when this decision was made. It was both ludicrous and heartbreaking.

When Alan approached Adele and asked her to join me in taking forward the value-based healthcare project she jumped at the chance. She recalls thinking that if she could improve the care for just one patient, she would be happy. I remember meeting Adele and feeling like I was being put under the microscope. She was intensely curious about clinical care and wanted to understand every detail about pathways of care and operational service delivery. She would grill me, often for hours, in those early days, and she wrote everything down in notebook after notebook.

Adele had a remarkable ability to get things done. She knew how to work the system and help me achieve the early aims of the projects we set for ourselves. Our complementary skill sets became important given that we did not have a lot of resources to play with. She is one of the most driven and hard-working managers I have ever worked with.

In December 2015 Adele and I boarded a plane to Boston to attend the Harvard course. We were accompanied by Mark Bowling, an accountant with an interest in costing, whom Alan had identified as an important addition to the team. The short course – taught by Professors Michael Porter and Bob Kaplan, giants of Harvard Business School – was the seminal programme on value-based healthcare. The three of us spent a lot of time together over the next five days, poring over the vast quantities of study material and talking about each other's perspectives on healthcare. We studied late into the night and rose early to memorize case studies on outcomes measurement and costing. We were desperate not to be caught out if we were singled out for questioning by the laser sharp Professor Porter.

We began to understand the depth of our ignorance about each other's worlds and even how we interpreted language in different ways. It made us realize the value of multiprofessional collaboration and how important this would be for the implementation of value-based healthcare. Alan had created the beginnings of a guiding coalition for value-based healthcare.[2]

Adele and I returned to the United Kingdom exhausted, but excited about how we were going to put the principles of value into practice. I knew that we were operating in a different context to that in the United States, but I was convinced that the principles of value – achieving the outcomes that matter to people while reducing or maintaining costs – were universally applicable. We just needed to figure out how to make that stick in Wales.

Shortly after we returned from the course, Adele and I had an opportunity to broaden our knowledge of the concept of value in health. We spotted a conference in Oxford intriguingly named 'Hellish Decisions in Healthcare'. It was convened by Professor Sir Muir Gray, who had written extensively on the concept of value in healthcare in the European context and was one of the contributors to an important European Commission report on value-based healthcare.[3]

Like the Harvard course, this short conference had a profound influence on my thinking at the time. Firstly, from my perspective, Muir's work on value was very relevant to Wales as it complemented Porter and Teisberg's work in the context of publicly funded universal healthcare systems. This was particularly true of the emphasis on population health and 'allocative value', i.e. how we apportion resources across whole pathways of care to get the best outcomes.[4] Secondly, the conference gave me my first opportunity to learn about the impressive work done on outcome data variation by the Scuola Superiore Sant'Anna in Pisa, Italy.

The relevant conference presentation was given by Professor Sabina Nuti, who subsequently became the rector of this highly selective public research university. The university had been gathering clinical outcome data from Italian states for more than 20 years, and they present variation data publicly on their website across multiple patient pathways.

Professor Nuti's presentation concerned a piece of work in the field of diabetes in which adverse outcome data (amputation rates, in this case) had been compared across participating states and significant variation demonstrated. Clinical teams were brought together to understand this variation, after which significant improvements were seen. It struck me how effective these clinical networks were in coming together around the data and finding what was driving good and bad outcomes. Just as striking was the quality of the data visualization in allowing assimilation of large amounts of information in an instant. I have yet to find more effective techniques to display complex sets of variation in healthcare.[5]

The final golden nugget from the 'Hellish' conference was a talk by the German psychologist Professor Gerd Gigerenzer. The topic was uncertainty and risk, and specifically how we react to those things in the context of healthcare. As a general practitioner managing the risks of undifferentiated first presentations of illness daily, this was particularly fascinating. Many of our behaviours and actions as clinicians are driven by anxiety for our patients in the face of huge uncertainty. Uncertainty about diagnosis (which is frequently complex, and not straightforward as hindsight and algorithms would have us believe), uncertainty about outcomes, and fear of veering away from guidelines even when doing so is justified. We need shared ownership of that risk and uncertainty with all actors in healthcare, or at the very least we need empathy for the situation. Without that, all attempts at reducing unnecessary diagnostic tests or prescribing are doomed to fail. It reminded me of Mary T. Lathrap's great poem 'Judge Softly', and specifically a line that my father had quoted to me often: 'Take the time to walk a mile in his moccasins.'

I left Oxford thinking about how to put all of this together and about how huge a cultural shift was needed to edge us towards value in health.

Starting to conceptualize value-based healthcare

By early 2016 we were in the midst of the ICHOM partnership. Claude Pinnock had been assigned as our project manager to support outcomes measurement in Parkinson's disease clinics. We were mapping out the patient pathway with Alastair Church (a neurologist) and Debbie Davies (a clinical nurse specialist) in St Woolos clinic in Newport. It was clear that implementing patient-reported outcome measures (PROMs) in practice was going to be a very large undertaking – one I will describe in more detail in chapter 4. I will forever be grateful to Alastair and Debbie for their tenacity and patience with us, and also to Claude, who went onto bigger and better things and became a chief medical officer in New York.

In addition to our work on outcomes, we were reflecting on all that we had alredy learned: from our time in Harvard, from Muir's work and conference, and from ICHOM. I thought that we needed a way of bringing this all together and a more strategic approach to our growing programme of work, much of which involved engagement with clinical teams and explaining the ethos of what we were trying to do. My first rather crude attempt at conceptualizing the required elements of value-based healthcare is seen in figure 1.

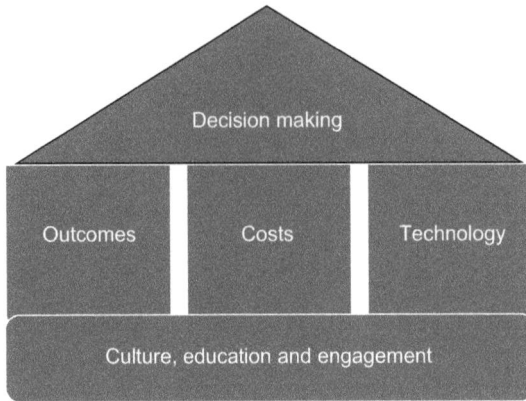

Figure 1. An early model for the implementation of value-based healthcare in the Aneurin Bevan Health Board.

This basic conceptual model was intended to illustrate the importance of cultural change and continued multiprofessional education and engagement as an underpinning necessity for successful value-based healthcare implementation. The three pillars represent the need to build internal infrastructure and capability to measure outcomes and costs. This includes the procurement of patient-facing technology to communicate digitally with people and capture patient-reported outcomes. Finally, the decision-making 'roof' highlights the need to use the data to support decision making towards better outcomes, whether that is clinical decision making in the therapeutic consultation or organizational investment in new services, technologies or patient support.

Progress towards value-based healthcare: three tests

The development of our conceptual model was helpful in keeping us on track and in developing our work plan to drive value-based healthcare in the organization, but I knew it was not going to be enough. The attempt to change culture was a lot of effort. Adele and I both spent a lot of time in the coffee shop in the Royal Gwent Hospital in Newport, meeting with clinical colleagues to talk about value-based healthcare. We soon realized we needed a more systematic approach to communications, education and engagement. We knew we needed to understand our outcomes and costs, of course, and we were beginning to see that if we were to scale up patient-reported outcome measurement, we would need patient-facing technology to help us cope with the larger volumes of communication and data. Finally, we knew that even if we managed to create belief in this approach and had data to drive value-based decision making, it would still come to nothing if we were unable to influence value-based decision making in either the consulting room or the boardroom.

Despite our progress and the growing support from clinical colleagues, I was still worried we would lose momentum. Health organizations are notoriously impatient for results, and value-based care is a long-term systemic shift. It became imperative to think about some shorter-term gains and to introduce some internal tests to see if the organization could start to move in a value-based healthcare direction. To my mind, we needed to achieve three things:

- demonstrate the impact of measuring patient-reported outcomes and establish it as a worthwhile activity;

- convince the board to invest in patient-facing technology to collect outcomes; and

- demonstrably increase value across a single pathway.

I therefore privately set myself these internal tests as markers of successful progress.

We had begun to garner wide clinical support for outcome measurement, and we had discovered that, unbeknown to us, two of my clinical colleagues had participated in another ICHOM standard outcomes set development! Steph Gething (an occupational therapist) had contributed to the stroke set[6] and Dr Steve Hutchison (a cardiologist) had been involved with the development of the heart failure set.[7] This was a real boost.

We urgently needed software to scale up patient-reported outcomes capture, and we were able to convince the board without too much difficulty that we should proceed with the necessary procurement. This was an unusual situation, to say the least. I believe our success came down to a handful of key factors. The first was the board engagement that Alan had undertaken; the involvement of the non-executive directors meant that a culture of innovation had been allowed to flourish. Second, not only did the board have sufficient confidence in us, as a team, to make the work a success, but there was also a sense of optimism and pride about the partnership we had formed with ICHOM. We were allowed to proceed with a degree of uncertainty that would not normally have been entertained. We were given freedom to act and we were allowed to fail.

During this time we were immensely grateful for the support ICHOM gave us. The encouragement we were given helped us a great deal during the difficult days when we were realizing the enormity of the task ahead. The rigour that Thomas Kelley, ICHOM's vice president, brought to our project management was also deeply appreciated.

This all represented steady progress towards our goal of creating an outcomes-focused, value-based healthcare organization, but I knew we needed to demonstrate the value and impact of our work even before more outcome data became available. Leaving our existing programme management and the details of the software business case to Adele, I turned my attention to a clinical project and the challenging business of demonstrating increased value for patients across a whole pathway of care.

Demonstrating value across a whole pathway of care

Work on the chronic obstructive pulmonary disease (COPD) pathway in the Aneurin Bevan University Health Board had begun in late 2015. The pathway work was initiated in the primary care division because of a need to understand variation in prescribing patterns for the disease, and I was now chairing a multidisciplinary group comprising GPs, respiratory consultants, patients, pharmacists, operational managers and an accountant.

COPD is a debilitating chronic lung condition that causes breathlessness and exacerbations that frequently result in hospital admission. The mainstays of treatment are

- smoking cessation;
- immunization against common respiratory viruses, e.g. influenza and Covid-19;
- non-pharmacological support for symptom management, pulmonary rehabilitation and peer-group support; and
- inhaler therapy (including inhaled corticosteroids for more severe disease).

The impact on patient outcomes relative to cost is not uniform across these interventions, with inhaled therapy being far more costly per quality-adjusted life year (QALY).[8] There is particular uncertainty[9] about the addition of inhaled corticosteroids, and the National Institute for Health and Care Excellence (NICE) is very specific about their use in its guidelines for COPD.[10]

Our prescribing data showed that we were higher prescribers than one would expect based on our available prevalence and severity data (obtained from primary care coding). We also had one of the highest exacerbation and admission rates in Wales – a fact that was unexplained. Additionally, there was inequitable access to both pulmonary rehabilitation and peer support, and there was a lack of choice when it came to options for smoking cessation support. Patients and GPs alike reported that the growing number of new drugs and inhaler device types was causing inconsistency and confusion. There was a clear feeling that the inconsistency was causing suboptimal inhaler technique – something that is critical to proper drug delivery to the lung.

Considering these issues, the group was unanimous in its resolve.

- Formulary choices needed to be rationalized, with patients being able to choose their preferred inhaler device for each of the drug classes they were prescribed. This consistency would enable them to stick to mastering a single inhaler technique, thereby getting more from their medicine. The new pathway guidance needed to be embedded through continuing professional development (CPD) events for GPs and practice nurses and supported by consultant educational podcasts.

- A long-term plan to maintain high levels of competence in inhaler technique training was required.

- A business case needed to be developed for reinvesting potential prescribing savings into pulmonary rehabilitation and other non-pharmacological interventions.

Despite being an integrated care organization with oversight of the whole pathway, from prevention through to end-of-life care, I knew that the third of these three aims was going to be the most difficult to achieve. It was also the most value-based in its approach. I knew it had to succeed if we were serious about adopting value-based healthcare as a system, and I also knew I would have to resign if it failed. This was the case because it is not enough simply to understand the outcomes in our healthcare organizations: we also have a responsibility to understand how we are utilizing resources to achieve those outcomes and to make changes if what we are doing is suboptimal.

In Wales this meant overcoming the budgetary silos that existed between different organizational departments by creating a notional programme budget covering all the interventions needed by patients who were either at risk of or were being treated for a certain condition (or by a sub-population with similar needs, such as frail elderly people). In my view this is analogous to the idea of bundled payments[11] in insurance-based or other payment systems, the idea being that you link finance to everything that patients need across a whole pathway of care and optimize that through an analysis of outcomes. This has nothing to do with benchmarking for competition: it is about being transparent around outcomes and costs and creating a learning health and care system that seeks both to improve value for patients and to create sustainable healthcare systems for society. I was delighted that we had an accountant on the group who bought into this philosophy.

By March 2017 South East Wales had hugely improved the quality of prescribing in COPD and had significantly reduced the associated costs. It was now time to reinvest those savings in pulmonary rehabilitation to achieve equitable access to services across the region's five boroughs. I was thinking about Janice – my patient who we met in the book's introduction – as this was so similar to other chronic disease management scenarios.

We needed to boost non-pharmacological support alongside medicinal support medicines if we were to improve patient outcomes. I will not claim that this was easy. It almost failed because the savings were made from the primary care prescribing budget, which is entirely separate from the respiratory directorate budget that the new investment needed to come from. In the end, though, the board agreed to making it happen through an internal corporate finance mechanism made possible by the integrated health board status, meaning that we achieved our aim.

When value-based improvements were made to costs, either through improved outcomes or by reducing low-value activity, we found it critical to reinvest at least a proportion of that revenue into services for that same group of patients otherwise clinical teams became disillusioned and disengaged very quickly. In our context, this meant using corporate finance to adjust internal budgets and reinvest savings, whereas in competition-based and profit-driven systems, it means reinvestment of profit. Regardless, the same principle applies.

Clinical teams looking after a particular patient group are highly motivated to engage in hard work if the incentive is to deliver more for the patients they are caring for. This is something that the team at the Santeon Group of hospitals in the Netherlands also found, as evidenced by the following quote from their paper in the *NEJM Catalyst* journal:

> In addition to the technical challenges and administrative burden, Santeon did not directly reinvest the additional income generated by the value-based reimbursement contracts in the improvement teams that developed the value-based improvement initiatives that largely contributed to Santeon's efforts to meet value-based [key performance indicators (KPIs)]. This was unintentional but ultimately had a negative impact on motivation and long-term KPI compliance.[12]

The postscript to this story was that the pulmonary rehabilitation services went on to measure outcomes across the five models of care across the five boroughs, and time-driven, activity-based costing was also carried out. All of this helped us understand which was the highest-value model. The whole programme was a great success – a monument to the velvet bulldozers in the COPD group, who did not give up. I would have like to have seen this approach replicated far more often, but corporate structures are hard to budge.

A properly organized and resourced outfit: building the value-based healthcare programme

By this stage we had procured software that allowed us to scale patient-reported outcome measurement across the health board, and Adele had appointed a small project management team to help us meet the growing demand from clinical teams in the organization to get involved with value-based healthcare.

Although we had spent a lot of time on clinical and financial engagement, one of the mistakes we made was to fail to involve operational managers early enough in conversations. Very often, this important group had a different set of pressures and targets imposed on them. We soon learned that everything grinds to a halt without them so it was a lesson we had to learn quickly!

Everyone was under so much pressure. We needed a small team with dedicated time to support PROMs and other aspects of value-based healthcare implementation alongside clinical teams. In Adele's words, 'we needed to move from evangelism to being a properly organized and resourced outfit with a multidisciplinary approach'. Building internal organizational capability and capacity in value-based healthcare is essential for sustained scaling and impact.

Early forays into costing for value

When Mark Bowling returned from Harvard, Alan set him off on another proof of concept in parallel with the work that Adele and I were pursuing. Having secured agreement from the directors of finance of each of the health boards in Wales, Mark was given full access to clinical teams to undertake time-driven, activity-based costing[13] in all the cataract pathways of care. Initially this involved meeting with all of the clinical teams to map out each cataract pathway, including the number of steps and the costs associated with each step, including staff time. This was a very laborious exercise even for a relatively simple and short pathway of care such as cataract surgery.

Mark found a significant variation in cost (40% between the highest-cost and lowest-cost pathways) that was mostly down to a variation in the number of steps that patients had to go through in the pathway prior to surgery. Variation could be seen between organizations, with suboptimal utilization of optometry skills in the community, and there was also pathway variation between different ophthalmologists within a single hospital, e.g. in the number of steps in the pathway when patients were worked up for surgery. Mark's analysis highlighted the utility of this approach in identifying invisible costs that were not contributing to patient outcomes.

Interestingly, presentation of the variation in this data did not immediately produce significant change. I have reflected often about why this might have been. Perhaps because we did not yet have the outcome data presented alongside the costs? Perhaps because we had failed to present the data in the right way to the right people? Time-driven, activity-based costing is time consuming, and it is difficult to easily revisit the exercise without more internal costing resource. How could we streamline that process?

In tandem with Mark's cataract pathway analysis, we were participating in the Global Health Outcomes Benchmarking (GLOBE) programme[14] as one of ICHOM's strategic partners. This saw a number of ICHOM's international partners capturing clinical and patient-reported outcomes, which was a very laborious exercise at the time, involving manually transposing anonymized clinical and patient-reported outcome data into huge spreadsheets. At this point we were inching forwards as international collaborators on a challenging project that had never previously been attempted. The experience illustrated to us the importance of good healthcare information infrastructure (especially data interoperability) to make data capture easy as part of direct care.

Despite the challenges, this exercise enabled our entire cadre of ophthalmologists, under the leadership of Mr Chris Blyth, to compare their outcomes with each other and to understand what that comparison meant for their practice. Since that initial pilot, ICHOM has digitized and harmonized all its sets of measures, aligning them with international digital standards. As a result, it has now been able to set up the first true international learning collaborations, with solid technical standards as the backbone. This activity has also prompted huge development in the PROMs software market, with new products that have much-improved functionality and better attention to data models/interoperability.

Going national with value-based healthcare

By late 2017 value-based healthcare was becoming mainstream in the Aneurin Bevan Health Board and we were witnessing a degree of cultural shift towards outcome measurement, mainly in our hospitals. We had developed a strategy and a small but multiskilled programme team. Teams were starting to measure outcomes across fifteen or so clinical areas and inspiring stories of the difference this was making for patients were beginning to emerge. We seemed to be reaching a tipping point of engagement within the health board, but there was a problem. Value-based healthcare requires a focus on outcomes, costs and associated system mechanisms to drive greater value. Our organization was being driven by a different – government-provided – set of activity-based indicators and priorities, and if this did not change it was difficult to see how we could make further progress.

I was also coming to realize that value-based healthcare decision making required significant changes to the digital and data landscape across Wales. At that point I did not know if it would be possible to engage with the NHS Wales Informatics Service on this topic (the national organization responsible for digital services at that time). The dream of achieving a healthcare system based on decision making to improve the outcomes that mattered to patients seemed a long way off. We had reached the limits of our 'bottom-up' approach to value-based healthcare and we needed systemic obstacles to change or to be moved out of the way.

But then a breakthrough occurred. Alan was appointed as the director of finance for NHS Wales. It was time to go national.

In a short space of time Alan made a few key interventions. First, he established the Finance Academy to support the professional development of all finance professionals in Wales. He then created the Finance Delivery Unit to improve financial performance through the optimization of resource utilization. Both had the value-based healthcare philosophy at their core, with the idea being to embed value-based approaches in the finance community for the long term. At the same time Alan was in discussion with the chief medical officer to create a new clinical post: the National Clinical Director for Prudent and Value-Based Healthcare. I decided to go for it.

For a clinician, jumping into the policy arena is – at least initially – a bewildering experience. I had no idea how to get things done in that world, and despite still practising as a GP, I felt far removed from my colleagues in healthcare. I was also very sad to leave behind both Adele and the work we had been doing at the Aneurin Bevan Health Board, which was really taking off. Government was a lonely place to be, not least because for the first year I had no team and no resources to build one.

I set about building relationships and seeking permission to write a National Strategy for Value-Based Healthcare in Wales. Given that Wales already had a long-term strategy for health and care through the 'A healthier Wales' report, I had to settle for a three-year action plan.[15] Understanding how to be flexible in developing the aims within an existing policy framework was key learning for me, but I was still able to incorporate all the key elements that were needed to drive value-based healthcare nationally. The objectives for my proposed plan were drawn from the learning obtained from value-based healthcare implementation in the Aneurin Bevan University Health Board, and the plan was organized around six goals.

- **Goal 1. Working with patients.** Ensure that outcomes measurement is embedded as part of direct care to benefit patients immediately.

- **Goal 2. Health informatics and analytics.** Influence the digital transformation necessary to embed PROMs measurement in care, including the creation of dashboards and other information products for operational use.

- **Goal 3. Outcomes and costs.** Build the capacity and capability to implement cost and outcome measurement across Wales.

- **Goal 4. Communication, education and engagement.** Embed a culture of value across Wales through informal and formal education, growing a repository of case studies and other educational resources. For people to access education, they have to be engaged with a topic, and outreach to professional groups in all parts of the system therefore needs to continue in parallel.

- **Goal 5. Research and industry.** Work in partnership with academia and the life sciences industry to influence a move towards applying value-based principles in the adoption and use of medicines, medical devices and other technologies. Grow the value-based healthcare research base.

- **Goal 6. Strategic partnerships.** Continue to build national and international networks of organizations and individuals to create momentum in value-based healthcare culture change.

At a governmental level, there was a great need for cultural change towards measurement of and transparency around clinical and patient-reported outcomes, as well as building momentum around the aims of value-based healthcare to improve care for the people of Wales. As my resources were limited, I focused entirely on this in the early days: without garnering support, I would never gain the necessary funding to support implementation nationally. Once the programme started to gain momentum, my focus expanded to galvanizing everyone involved in the digital and data landscape in Wales to support a move towards the systematic capture and use of clinical and patient-reported outcomes. This was a monumental task.

Additionally, the chief medical officer asked me to contribute to his annual report,[16] which was to have value in health as its central theme.

Looking back, I believe that these interventions, along with ongoing and relentless communication and engagement with stakeholders from every discipline, were the factors that enabled me to secure a small budget. I now had the resources I needed to begin building a team and to achieve the primary goals.

Momentum was growing, thanks to successful engagement with the Finance Delivery Unit, the Finance Academy and my colleagues at the NHS Wales Informatics Service, notably Helen Thomas, the head of information at the time. By the summer of 2019 I had created a small team that was working in a loose matrix across several organizations. I had also commissioned a block contract with the NHS Wales Informatics Service to build an internal data team focused on value-based data infrastructure. This was to prove to be a key enabler for value-based healthcare in Wales. Alongside this I had secured a merger with another government-funded programme: the National PROMs, PREMs and Clinical Effectiveness Programme.

The nPROMs, as it was affectionately known, was a national project set up in 2016 by some far-sighted individuals at the

Cardiff and Vale University Health Board, who had secured fund-ing to measure PROMs through the Efficiency Through Tech-nology Fund (ETTF), a national innovation fund from the Welsh government. Interestingly, this was not linked to value-based healthcare as such, but was instead more akin to other large, centralized PROM collections such as the one commissioned by NHS England. In 2019 nPROMs was about to be defunded because the ETTF was being wound up, but I persuaded the decision makers to continue the programme by merging nPROMs with the value-based healthcare programme. Over-night, the merged programme acquired the expertise of Sarah Puntoni and Amanda Willacott, two experience PROMs pro-gramme managers. Their experience of PROMs implementation was later to prove pivotal to the development of the PROMs Standard Operating Model for Wales, something we will discuss in detail in chapter 7.

The other critical addition to the value programme from the old nPROMs was the PROMs team from CEDAR.[17] CEDAR is an independent research institute in Wales with wide-ranging expertise, including expert knowledge around PROMs selec-tion, translation and validation, licensing and analysis. Access to this type of expertise is critical to any organization or health-care system that wants to implement PROMs for the purpose of value-based healthcare, bringing those PROMs together with clinical outcome and other data for analysis.

In parallel with my acquisitions, Alan had arranged for two further health boards to have a small amount of funding spe-cifically to grow fledgling value-based healthcare teams in their organizations. This was designed to accelerate the move towards value-based healthcare across the system and it was very effective.

But then, Covid-19 arrived.

On 12 March 2020 I asked the team to redeploy themselves as they saw fit to support efforts to deal with the first wave of the pandemic. This crisis commanded all of our attention until the autumn of that year. The team came back together, virtually, in September 2020 to continue our work, albeit with an initial focus on data work centred around outcomes because of the impact of the pandemic. By January 2021 I was redeployed again, along with many of the team, into the vaccine campaign.

In July 2021 it was time to regroup. Alan was planning to retire and I was anxious both to secure a home for my team, who were scattered to the four winds, and to consolidate three separate budget streams. Alan convened a meeting with Ifan Evans, a government official, and Paul Mears, the CEO of Cwm Taf Morgannwg University Health Board. Ifan agreed to continue to sponsor the programme and Paul gave us a home – important gestures, for which I continue to be extremely grateful.

The Welsh Value in Health Centre was born, and with it came a new strategy that took account of all the progress and learning to date.[18] This was a highly significant turn of events in the value-based healthcare story in Wales. It meant that I was able to bring the team together and create an important sense of belonging, which was something we all needed after the trials of the pandemic. It was now much easier to manage the programme from a governance perspective, and this was important given that it was becoming obvious that the healthcare system had taken some severe knocks as a result of Covid-19. Outcomes in the population had worsened; healthcare professionals were tired and burned out; resourcing was very tight. This scenario was not unique to Wales, of course: it could be seen playing out all over the world.

After the pandemic, as a result of the establishment of the Value in Health Centre, the team and the work they were doing had a home and an international 'face'. The centre became a rallying point for many colleagues working in value-based healthcare globally. It was now an entity, and I hoped this would give it longevity.

There is no doubt in my mind that key to the early national wins in value-based healthcare were the goodwill and belief of a multiprofessional coalition of people in different organizations who had developed the same shared purpose: to pursue better outcomes and a more sustainable healthcare system. Even at the centre, bottom-up approaches came before structural change. The 'why' of value-based healthcare resonated deeply with many.

Key lessons from chapter 2

Leadership and strategic vision

Alan Brace's journey highlights the importance of boundary-spanning leadership that challenges conventional roles in healthcare, integrating clinical understanding with strategic financial management.

Collaboration with the International Consortium for Health Outcomes Measurement (ICHOM) was crucial in supporting early implementation through giving us the confidence and expertise to project manage early outcomes measurement, but it was vital to build internal capability beyond that first phase. External validation from credible institutions like ICHOM helps maintain momentum.

Building a guiding coalition

The early formation of a small but committed coalition helped drive change, ensuring key stakeholders from both the clinical and executive levels were engaged. Sponsorship and support from senior figures is necessary if obstacles are to be overcome.

Cultural change and multiprofessional collaboration

Long-term cultural change is needed in healthcare. This must include tackling the often-adversarial relationship between the clinical and managerial worlds. Different perspectives, coming together, are a powerful force for effective change. If clinical teams are to remain engaged in value-based healthcare, incentives are necessary. These do not need to be incentives for personal gain: they can instead relate to investment of new revenues into the patients that are being caring for.

The transition from local success in the Aneurin Bevan Health Board to a national strategy for Wales required structural and policy changes.

Challenges and adaptability

While the Covid-19 pandemic put an initial pause on progress, it also reinforced the need for value-based healthcare because of the heightened focus on improving outcomes and sustainability. As a result, we saw a re-emergence and acceleration of our work.

The establishment of entities such as the Welsh Value in Health Centre ensure long-term sustainability for value-based healthcare initiatives.

CHAPTER 3

A gentle revolution from within

'You cannot buy the revolution. You cannot make the revolution. You can only be the revolution. It is in your spirit or it is nowhere.'
— Ursula K. Le Guin, *The Dispossessed* (1974)

Shifting the culture in healthcare: how to build a movement

Evolving healthcare so that it meets the changing needs of our populations around the world requires a radical shift in the way we think about system and service structures, governance, funding and even the roles of healthcare professionals. It certainly requires a radical shift in the way that professionals think about interacting with patients – and in how patients think about interacting with them.

It is hard for us to reimagine healthcare delivery because we are all hardwired to think and operate in a certain way, whether we are a patient, a politician, a clinician, a manager or an accountant. This can sometimes stifle our imagination when it comes to doing things differently, or it can cause us to pour more and more resources into futile attempts at service sustainability. In the United Kingdom, this might manifest itself as tired planning mechanisms that focus on short-term fixes to increase the number of appointments or procedures that get carried out (increasing productivity, in other words). In taxation-funded systems such as the NHS in Wales, an example would be costly interventions to reduce outpatient waiting times without reviewing patients' needs and then designing innovative solutions to meet those needs in the community. In private hospitals, where making a profit is a driver for healthcare delivery, there might be a push to increase the number of patients and procedures because the organization is paid for the activity. The key point is that neither scenario pays attention to whether the increased productivity actually improves patient outcomes or considers whether there was a lower-cost way of achieving the desired outcome. In other words, we can never make a complete analysis of productivity in healthcare unless we measure outcomes and costs.

Value-based healthcare offers a way of looking at the way we do things with fresh eyes. It requires us to assess the status quo critically, using outcome, process and cost data to inform how we redesign services to meet patients' needs in a sustainable fashion. Early on in our work on value-based healthcare in Wales it became clear that culture change – through the education and engagement of colleagues around these principles and ways of working – was critical to any chance we had of success. The theory and the technical details about why value-based healthcare is important are one thing, but no large transformational change will occur without culture change happening first. Changing the culture in healthcare is a mammoth task; it requires a revolution from within. If you are trying to create such a change, you must demonstrate that you really believe in it, you must stand up for that belief, and you need to be prepared to take criticism and challenge with good humour. You must be credible.

For culture change to occur, there must be underlying dissatisfaction at the way things are. In the early twenty-first century, there is a prevailing sense that all is not well in healthcare, and that we cannot continue along current trajectories. In short, we have a burning platform for change.[1]

In the early days of the value-based healthcare work in the Aneurin Bevan University Health Board, my attempts to recruit people to our cause consisted mainly of talking to colleagues at length over cups of coffee. I was fortunate to have a broad network of people I had collaborated with. They came from several different areas of work and from across the spectrum of hospital-based, primary and community care. There was a degree of trust between us that meant that while I was initially regarded with scepticism by some, I was not immediately shown the door. I did have to buy a lot of cake and coffee in the hospital cafe, however. The importance of engaging (and recruiting) my colleagues was paramount to me.

Over time, I began to put some structure and purpose behind the work of communication, education and engagement, and this later formed a key pillar in the national strategy. Indeed, this work continues even as the technical work of outcomes-driven care reform starts to take shape and bear fruit. One of my favourite YouTube videos about creating a social movement is the clip of the 'Dancing Man', in which a lone man starts to do some crazy moves on a sunny hillside at a music festival. He is surrounded by groups of people who initially watch his dancing with bemusement. Then one other guy joins him, mirroring the crazy moves. Before too long, the entire hillside of festival-goers are involved. This vignette is a brilliant metaphor for creating a followership: a critical mass of people willing to do the work with you because they believe in it too.[2]

Make no mistake, this work is painstaking and it takes time. In the early days of our project, the subject was very new, its aims seemed impossible, and many clinicians were suspicious that it would be just another cost-cutting or finger-pointing exercise about performance management. They understood the need for stewardship of resources but they wanted some reciprocity from the system to support improvement in outcomes for their patients. Building trust across professional boundaries was of critical importance, and the way to build that trust was through demonstrating integrity. We had to show both that we would follow through on supporting teams to measure outcomes and that promises would be kept around the allocation of resources to new value-based care models, to give two important examples.

My feeling was that the key to building the movement was to get some respected senior clinical colleagues on board first. That meant carefully allocating the necessary time, care and effort to work around their diaries, to do the required legwork, to understand the pressures they were under – and to buy more cake.

As individual conversations grew into seminars and group presentations, language became increasingly important. Each new presentation on value-based healthcare was bespoke to the people I was speaking to. This meant that, five years into the project, I had several hundred presentation decks. They all had a slightly different flavour to enable me to get into other people's worlds, to engage with them and to build trust.

Sometimes I did not even use the term value-based healthcare at the outset. This did not mean that I was veering away from the principles of value-base healthcare, just that it is often better to avoid jargon and the threat of misunderstanding until common ground and trust are achieved. People who work in healthcare are usually very busy, and they are generally working under a lot of pressure. If you want to persuade them to support a cause, they need to know it is immediately relevant to their context and that it is going to be helpful to their aims and objectives in caring for patients. You must enter their world and let them know what is in it for them.

Surprisingly, perhaps, momentum grew rapidly. The emerging ethos of a focus on outcomes as a driver for trans-formational change in the health board seemed to resonate with both clinicians and accountants alike. As the movement towards value-based healthcare grew, I had to take great care to ensure that the approach was not seen as a new paradigm for overthrowing others that were already in play – notably, the quality-improvement community, health economists engaged in cost-effectiveness analyses, and the architects of prudent healthcare. I was keen for all of us to work together. High-value care, i.e. care that improves the outcomes that really matter to people while also addressing the optimal use of resources to achieve them, has a number of prerequisites. These include quality-improvement methodologies and health technology assessments as vital contributors to value in health, but these are insufficient to achieve value on their own. The relationship between value, quality and health technology assessments will be examined in more detail later in the book.

Making approaches to try to engage separate – but related – camps might seem like a trivial matter, but it is not. Doing so is essential to achieving a critical mass of support, which is needed to influence a national change of direction in policy towards a focus on outcomes and value-based healthcare. Porter and Teis-berg's original theory of value-based healthcare suggested that outcomes (and value) would only be improved through com-petition between clinicians, providers and systems, but what I discovered, as we explored implementation, was that while we needed to capture and compare outcomes, value-based healthcare was far more likely to succeed through collaboration across healthcare pathways rather than through market-based competition between organizations.

There is a caveat to this statement, though, and that is that if we are going to see outcomes improve and value increase, we must be transparent with our data. Every healthcare system needs a mindset of improvement and a willingness to learn. This means we must face up to failings at times as well as celebrating successes. Failure to be transparent is failing patients.

Clinical culture, part 1

Certain clinical tribes bought into value-based healthcare – and particularly the use of patient-reported outcomes – very quickly. In fact, some were already using PROMs in the direct care of their patients, but were not necessarily describing that activity in the context of value-based healthcare. Allied health professionals such as physiotherapists, speech and language therapists and audiologists were in the vanguard. The other professional group leading the way were clinical nurse specialists. This latter group were early pioneers in Wales, working in the fields of lung cancer, heart failure and lymphoedema.[3,4]

Driving a cultural shift in healthcare is a relentless, never-ending task. It is a task so complex and huge that even the analogy of turning an oil tanker around is insufficient to describe its magnitude. It is more like persuading wildebeest to alter their migratory path across the Serengeti.

As interest in value-based healthcare as a hopeful vehicle for change began to grow, individual meetings over coffee gave way to more formal requests for seminars and workshops by clinical departments in the health board, professional societies and our sponsoring executive board. Early seminars were not always plain sailing. I remember a particularly challenging joust at a meeting of the Welsh Cardiological Society at which I was told that the clinical outcome data quoted in my presentation was 'rubbish' as it was of poor quality. The data in question had been drawn from the published NHS Wales cardiovascular atlas of variation.[5] I gently reminded the hecklers that as this was our data, it was our collective duty to improve its quality, and that was only going to happen if we shone a light on it and used it to improve outcomes. My audience were not impressed.

I was not encountering a lack of interest in outcome data here though, simply frustration at the lack of infrastructure and organizational support for reliably capturing clinical outcome data and input into audits and registries. This was in stark contrast to the capture of process or financial data, and on this point I shared my colleagues' frustration intensely. I have never understood, and will never understand, the mismatch of attention given to different types of vital information in healthcare systems. There is a lack of parity of esteem between administrative data and clinical or patient-reported data. This is particularly true of financial data. If we are to make progress towards higher-value healthcare, this situation has to change.

We adjourned for dinner and, thankfully, for more amicable conversations. The cardiologists present were supportive of the value-based healthcare philosophy but highly sceptical that progress would be made to support its implementation at scale.

Getting senior leaders on board: the importance of powerful sponsorship

When Alan moved from his role as director of dinance in the Aneurin Bevan University Health Board to the same role for NHS Wales, he drove further action to accelerate the adoption of value-based healthcare across Wales.

First, he brokered an expansion of the ICHOM partnership to involve the other health boards in the measurement of outcomes. The plan was to begin with lung cancer. This venture was not as successful as we had hoped, probably because there was not yet a readiness within the other boards to drive forward the wider cultural and organizational change needed to embed outcome measurement in care. For a start, there was a lack of patient-facing technology, so the other health boards had to use the data platform built by the NHS Wales Informatics Service (NWIS) for the National PROMs, PREMs and Clinical Effectiveness Programme (nPROMs). This platform had been built as a separate endeavour to enable the collection of PROMs according to the ICHOM-recommended time points in the pathway; it had not been designed for use in direct care, and this had a negative impact on its usability for both patients and clinicians.

It was not all bad news, however. The lung cancer team in Hywel Dda University Health Board out in rural West Wales really bought into the idea – and they were willing to persevere with the clunky technology. This meant that we began to have enough data to design prototype PROM data dashboards in the Welsh Clinical Portal, the nearest thing we had to a hospital electronic health record (EHR) at the time. It also paved the way for the first national outcome data dashboard to be created in lung cancer. Even though this information product did not have full national PROM data coverage, it began to attract the interest of the informatics community. Value-based healthcare began to be a useful vehicle for showcasing the data work and aspirations of NWIS (and later of Digital Health and Care Wales, which NWIS later became).

It could be said, therefore, that despite the national ICHOM project not achieving success in its initial objective of all organizations measuring patient-reported outcomes in lung cancer, it was not a total disaster. We had been allowed to fail, but in so doing we had engaged one team and we had learned a great deal more about data standards and user requirements for patient-facing technology. Most importantly, though, the digital and data community were on board and were getting behind value-based healthcare strategically. I was learning that multi-professional collaboration and boundary-spanning leadership were essential to effecting large-scale change. This was not just about clinicians and financial managers – everyone had a role to play.

Gaining senior sponsorship in the digital arena is pivotal to developing the infrastructure that is needed for value-based healthcare, whether that is support for procuring software, for defining and implementing data standards, for providing advice on information governance matters, or for building analytical tools. I quickly became enmeshed in the digital world. Later, when I had secured investment for a national value-based healthcare programme and team, I commissioned the appointment of an internal value-based healthcare team within NWIS with the full support of Helen Thomas, their director of information at that time. The number and diversity of value-based healthcare sponsors nationally was growing.

Alan Brace was keen to accelerate progress and capitalize on early wins. He was already in talks with the two health boards in West Wales – the Abertawe Bro Morgannwg University Health Board (now the Swansea Bay UHB) and Hywel Dda University Health Board – about resourcing fledgling value-based healthcare teams there to mirror the one that Adele and I had built. This turned out to be the game changer we needed to grow the value-based healthcare movement across Wales. Why not resource all boards to do this, you may ask? Well, I think Alan was being a little mischievous here and creating some competition and 'fear of missing out' in the boards at executive level! The medical director in Swansea at the time was Hamish Laing. Hamish was a keen advocate for value-based healthcare approaches, and his involvement was soon to become highly significant.

Setting up formal education: accelerating change through learning

As the value-based healthcare movement grew, it became clear that we needed a more systematic approach to value-based healthcare education in the region. Engagement meetings over cake and coffee and seminars to professional societies and within Welsh government were no longer meeting the demand that was there for knowledge about value-based healthcare and its implementation. Sadly, we could not send everyone to Harvard!

Additionally, learning needs were expanding and diversifying. Many people wanted access to entry-level learning into the basic theoretical basis for value-based healthcare. This meant that standardization was urgently required to ensure we avoided misinterpretation or misappropriation of what we were trying to achieve. Expanding the approaches to disseminating theoretical knowledge was not enough, however. There was now an appetite from teams to understand what this would mean for them on the ground, and how they could begin to put theory into practice. Action learning sets were developed by the Finance Academy and by the Hywel Dda health board. Both programmes were pedagogically accredited and focused on practical learning alongside a value-based healthcare project. Typically, a dyad of a clinician and an operational or finance manager did this together.

The most significant milestone in creating high-quality learning in value-based healthcare in Wales and beyond was the creation of the Intensive Learning Academy at Swansea University School of Management.[6] It was fortuitous that 'A healthier Wales', the long-term strategy for health and social care in Wales, already described the intent to create Intensive Learning Academies, with the aim of training the entire workforce in transformation and improvement of healthcare delivery. Tactical use of existing policy hooks was an extremely effective approach to driving value-based healthcare forward at a national level.

Now that value-based healthcare was gaining momentum as a driving force for change at a policy level, it was possible to influence the educational direction and content of one of the academies to be created. This is how the Intensive Learning Academy for Value-Based Health and Care was conceived, and it found its home in Swansea University's School of Management in the beautiful beachside Bay Campus under the leadership of Professor Hamish Laing.

Hamish Laing: leading the way on value-based healthcare education and procurement

Hamish Laing is a restorative plastic surgeon by trade, having established the Welsh sarcoma service. He loved the practical, problem-solving nature of the discipline and its variety. He describes plastic surgery as being a 'toolbox of solutions for the whole body and all ages'. He rapidly extended these problem-solving skills into medical management roles and was medical director in Swansea when Alan Brace made his move west in expanding the value-based healthcare vision for Wales.

Hamish was quick to embrace the opportunity to implement value-based healthcare in his health board, and recalled having a lightbulb moment in 2013 as he listened to Maureen Bisognano speak at the International Forum for Quality and Safety in Healthcare in London.

Maureen, now president emerita at the Institute for Health Improvement, was explaining that we should really stop asking patients 'What is the matter?' and instead ask them 'What matters to you?' It was a powerful speech and it made an impression on me as well, though Hamish and I had not yet met at this point. He tested Maureen's approach out on the next patient he saw in clinic. Jim was 43 and a builder. He had a large sarcoma in his leg and Hamish was planning to operate. Jim looked overwhelmed by the situation as Hamish explained the surgery. Then Hamish asked Jim: 'What really matters to you now?' Jim's reply was surprising: 'What matters to me today is that I promised to build my neighbour a wall next week and I don't want to let him down. Would it affect me if I delayed the surgery by one week?' Hamish was amazed. He had assumed that Jim would want surgery immediately and he was therefore pulling out all the stops to achieve that aim.

'Of course we can delay,' said Hamish. 'It won't affect the outcome at all.' Jim instantly relaxed, and the two of them finished planning the next steps. The episode had changed

Hamish's practice forever, and it had got him thinking about patient outcomes.

So when Alan met with Hamish about value-based health-care in 2017, Hamish was ready to take it on. Not only had he seen how it could benefit his own patients, but he saw it as a lens through which to tackle healthcare's seemingly intractable problems.

By the end of 2017 Hamish had been approached to establish the Intensive Learning Academy for Value-Based Health and Care at Swansea University Management School. Early in this work he became very interested in the implications of value-based healthcare for the life sciences industry. He was conscious that we needed to find new ways of financing high-cost medicines and devices as the current procurement approach was unsustainable. He was frustrated at the lack of a problem-solving mindset and, as a result, he has become a pioneer in promoting value-based procurement using patient outcome data.

Given that, in a properly integrated system, health and social care needs should be met seamlessly for patients, there was a desire to expand the learning to the social care workforce. As a result, the academy was named the Intensive Learning Academy for Value-Based Health and Care.

Popular executive education courses were developed quickly. The academy funding included scholarships for NHS staff. When learners were asked about the most enriching aspects of the short courses, they commented on its multi-disciplinary appeal, with clinicians, managers, financial managers and informaticians attending and working together. As we have already seen, the bringing together of different perspectives from the clinical, financial, data, policy and industrial worlds is critical to the successful implementation of value-based healthcare. The course content is particularly strong in defining high-value whole pathways of care (from prevention through to end-of-life care) and in working with industry/ value-based procurement.

The academy quickly expanded its offering to include a master's degree, a doctorate in business administration, and a portfolio of teaching case studies and research.

Despite having now moved into academia as a full-time professor, Hamish was keen that the work of the academy remained close to clinical practice and that the learning there was a stepping stone to implementation. The academy therefore came to develop three crucial interdependent functions: education, research and consultancy.

Later on, Hamish and I established a memorandum of understanding between the academy and the Welsh Value in Health Centre with a view to a longstanding partnership to do two things: first, to support the development of value-based healthcare in the Welsh NHS; and second – and importantly – to grow the network of international collaborators in the fields of education, clinical implementation and procurement.

Clinical culture, part 2: the creation of clinical networks

If we are to create long-term sustained change in the prevailing culture of healthcare delivery systems, we must grow the movement and keep up momentum. Otherwise, we will see regression.[7] Just as in the YouTube's 'Dancing Man', we must pass the leadership mantle to others. Pretty quickly, ad hoc engagement with individuals and small groups becomes insufficient to create sustained change and comes with the danger of misinterpretation of the message – or worse, misappropriation of the message. This is particularly true of value-base healthcare, where misappropriation can result in too much focus being placed on cost cutting or on redefining what is meant by an outcome that matters. Both of those things damage the mission reputationally and hamper progress towards true value for patients and healthcare organizations.

At this stage of implementation, we must systematize the approach to cultural change, and that means embedding it in the DNA of mainstream health policy and delivery mechanisms. Early in my role as national clinical director for value-based healthcare this was a real conundrum as I wrestled to garner coordinated policy support. Then I had a lucky break.

I received a call from a colleague, Dr Allan Wardhaugh, who had recently been appointed by the chief medical officer for Wales to devise a National Clinical Framework for Wales.[8] The framework was to be the blueprint for service redesign and was to cover optimal end-to-end clinical pathway design, including optimal staffing models and regionalization of specialist services. Allan, affectionately known as 'Sweary Al', is a straight-talking Scot; we hit it off straight away. Sitting in a Cardiff coffee shop on a cold January day in 2019, Allan told me that he was convinced that the National Clinical Framework should be constructed on value-based principles.

During the research and consultation phase for the National Clinical Framework, Allan and colleagues had noticed some clear themes arising.

1. The need to empower patients.

2. The need for a focus on improving outcomes and data-driven decision making.

3. The harms of 'too much medicine',[9] inequalities in health and unwarranted variation in care.

National clinical directors were already employed by government to advise on specific clinical policies related to their specialist areas, but they were frequently working in isolation and had little power to influence improvements in care on their own. The effect of this was that policy was handed to the seven health boards in Wales and enacted in seven different ways – this created a lot of variation in care, much of it unwarranted. It was increasingly obvious that we needed a coordinating mechanism to generate clinical consensus on standardized, evidence-based, whole-pathway approaches to care. The concept of clinical networks was born.

Allan Wardhaugh: a pioneering approach to clinical leadership

Allan trained as a general practitioner but re-entered hospital medicine due to his interest in paediatrics. He worked for a time at the prestigious Great Ormond Street Hospital in London as a paediatric intensivist. There, he was constantly immersed in high-tech care and was one of the pioneers of Picanet, the clinical registry for paediatric intensive care in the United Kingdom.

I asked Allan how he had come to be interested in broader philosophical thinking about modern medical practice and especially about value-based healthcare as a lens through which we could design better care. He told me that in paediatric intensive care he and his colleagues were dedicated to saving the lives of babies and children and improving the quality of life of these children and their families. He noticed there was a growing prevalence of technology-dependent children in PICU (the paediatric intensive care unit), some of whom did not survive their illness. The Picanet data demonstrated a clear trend that those that did not survive were having increasingly long lengths of stay in hospital before their death. He worried that instead of using technology to save lives as they intended, the decision making was instead resulting in prolonged suffering with no impact on outcome. This made him deeply uncomfortable and led to a desire to gain a much better understanding of patient outcomes to inform better decision making about interventions with families. A value-based healthcare seed had been planted in Allan's brain.

Some years later Allan was applying for a senior medical leadership role and was doing some background research in preparation for his interview. He recalls reading up about value-based healthcare and feeling like he was having an epiphany. He realized that there was language and a body of work to explain how clinical practice felt to him – and how it needed to change.

Allan's background as a paediatric intensivist and a clinical information officer with general practitioner training meant that he had a rare breadth of knowledge of the system and was a systems thinker. He understood what we were trying to achieve with value-based healthcare, and he appreciated the data requirements and national information architecture that would be needed to support the approach.

It was envisaged that clinical networks would describe 'ideal' care models to health boards and become part of the accountability process to reduce unwarranted variation in care. Key to this was the embedding of outcomes measurement, and in general a more systematic use of data for decision making. During the creation of the National Clinical Framework, Allan had heard a talk from the CEO of Intermountain Health in the United States in which a 'Learning Health System' was described.[10] This codified the thinking around a cycle of data-driven and value-based continuous improvement across the system: data to knowledge to practice and back to data again. Allan was keen to embed the concept of a Learning Health System in the National Clinical Framework. Further, he was explicit about including clinical and patient-reported outcome data in the datasets needed to drive continuous improvement in the system. This added futher weight to the Welsh Value in Health Centre's aims to improve the outcome data infrastructure in Wales, and specifically to drive investment in the technology and change management support needed to embed outcomes measures in care.

Thirteen networks were created, covering most of the disease burden in the population. The description of the value-based Learning Health System and the creation of the clinical networks systematized clinical engagement and a multiprofessional cultural shift towards value-based healthcare. This, combined with the engagement of the data community and the creation of formal learning, was the tipping point towards the wholesale cultural shift towards value-based healthcare in Wales.

Engaging patients and the public: champions of the cause

Patient and public engagement is, of course, vitally important to the implementation of value-based healthcare. This is not just about engagement in relation to the capture and use of patient-reported outcomes in support of care, though that is a cultural shift for patients too. The public also need to know about the 'crises' in healthcare[11] if they are to support their clinicians and health organizations in the noble pursuit of value in health, and even to lobby policymakers for change when the central levers for value-based healthcare are misaligned or weak.

This type of engagement plays out differently at local and organizational levels compared with the national landscape. For example, at the Aneurin Bevan University Health Board during the early days of the value-based healthcare programme, patients were very involved at a service level. Key patient representatives from each of the condition areas we were working on were instrumental in championing the benefits of outcome measurement and informing service improvements, e.g. in the heart failure and Parkinson's disease clinics.

Patient representatives contributed to videos we made about outcomes implementation, and they joined panel discussions at conferences. They were true champions of the work, often making progress with engagement where we found it difficult.

Nationally, the Welsh Value in Health Centre worked generically with patient charities and other national patient organizations, both to raise awareness of the ethos of value-based healthcare and to highlight its benefits for patients. The team also worked with patient groups on specific topics. For example, from the outset we had an excellent working relationship with Crohn's & Colitis UK, collaborating with them on several educational webinars and self-management resources for patients.[12]

Patient and public involvement at a national level was also imperative for the implementation of the PaRIS survey, which was run for Wales by the Welsh Value in Health Centre. This survey was a huge international initiative instigated by the Organisation for Economic Cooperation and Development (OECD) to measure the health outcomes and experiences of patients with chronic conditions treated in primary care settings. More details about the survey can be found in chapter 6.[13]

Engaging the world beyond: using professional communication to drive the mission forward

As far as the world is concerned, if you do not write about something, it did not happen. In the early days of value-based healthcare I was so immersed in the *doing* – of trying to make difficult changes happen – that I had no time or inclination to write much about it, still less to publish. Instead, I used Twitter to talk about the ideas and principles of value-based healthcare and about the problems I was seeing in the health system and how they might be addressed.

At that time, Twitter was a great social media platform both for building a network of like-minded people and also for floating more challenging or provocative ideas to change the status quo. Between 2014 and 2021, the platform was an incredibly powerful tool for supporting the creation of the social movement behind value-based healthcare as it enabled free ideas to flow freely between all the actors involved in healthcare, and it was especially good for involving patients, who, for the first time, could respond directly to professionals in a very transparent exchange of views. It also exposed me to more and more ideas, and it created a diverse international network that endures and grows to this day, even if Twitter's moment feels like it has passed. Social media remains an essential tool to build on progress in value-based healthcare, though – professionally, LinkedIn has assumed greater importance in promoting value-based healthcare, but it lacks the breadth of patient and public input I used to value so highly in Twitter's heyday.

I appointed a communications director to the team early in the development of the national work. The portfolio of work falling under the pillar of comms, education and engagement was one of the most important areas of focus in creating large-scale momentum. It came to include a range of products in support of our aims, both formal and informal. The website, case studies, conferencing, annual reports and animations to explain outcome measurement and implementation were all essential tools for driving forward our cultural mission.

Most popular of all was our 'health cast'. This monthly webinar always ran at the same time on a Friday lunchtime. The hope was that this would mean we could create something of a habitual institution that would stick in people's minds. The sessions, which covered a range of topics, were chaired by grassroots clinicians and value-based healthcare managers. Audience participation was encouraged, and sessions were recorded for sharing on YouTube.[14]

It is impossible to impose and implement value-based healthcare from the centre. The role of the centre should be to set policy and create enabling environments for value-based healthcare. This is likely to include the mandating of outcomes measurement and the creation of financial levers. Value-based healthcare implementation must be supported locally, with pods of professionals comprising clinical, managerial, financial and digital disciplines, and it needs to be embedded in organizational strategy.

By 2021 all health boards in Wales had their own value-based healthcare team coordinating their own programmes of work. These teams were brought together in a community of practice that was eventually formalized into the National Value-Based Healthcare Delivery Group. This group was pivotal in driving forward improvements in many areas, including the implementation of nationally agreed standard outcome sets and the PROMs standard operating model for Wales. They were also instrumental in supporting the design of new value-based care models in their organizations.

Several of the value-based healthcare leads from the health boards also supported the national work, by chairing the health cast, for example, or by providing material for case studies and chairing the PROMs Collaborative, a group established to ensure the appropriate use of PROMs at a national level and to share learning on implementation.

Key lessons from chapter 3

Systemic shifts

Radical shifts in thinking are required to evolve healthcare systems and meet the world's evolving population needs. This includes rethinking governance, funding, professional roles and patient interactions.

Cultural transformation precedes large-scale systemic change. A failure to address ingrained attitudes and behaviours will mean that any progress will soon peter out. Leadership must be federated to sustain and evolve the work – you must let go of your baby.

Reciprocity and the building of trust are essential to overcoming resistance, especially when introducing new frameworks like value-based healthcare. It is imperative that you do what you say you are going to do (following through for the long game) and not use the data for punitive ends.

Engaging stakeholders through personalized communication

Effective engagement involves speaking to people using language that resonates with them. Avoid jargon and make the message relevant to the purpose, context and challenges of your audience.

Building relationships with senior clinical leaders and tailoring approaches to different audiences creates the necessary momentum for change. For example, informal discussions over coffee can eventually evolve into structured seminars and presentations.

Creating a social movement

Change requires a critical mass of support. Influencing colleagues and building a network of advocates (or a 'followership') is painstaking but necessary work.

Collaboration, rather than competition, accelerates progress in value-based healthcare. The Welsh case study at the heart of this book has demonstrated the importance of avoiding divisive paradigms while aligning diverse groups such as health economists, quality improvement teams and clinicians. However, a collaborative approach should not give way to a lack of rigour. The way to improve care is through transparency of outcome data.

Leadership, collaboration and infrastructure

Sponsorship and leadership from key senior and multidisciplinary figures were pivotal in scaling value-based healthcare efforts in Wales.

Sustained change requires aligning clinical, managerial and digital leadership, supported by robust technology infrastructure and shared goals.

Initiatives such as clinical networks help to align goals across the system, to embed value-based healthcare principles in organizational DNA, and to create a culture of improvement in outcomes.

Education as a catalyst for change

Educational initiatives such as Swansea University's Intensive Learning Academy provide structured, multidisciplinary learning opportunities to advance national and international understanding of value-based health and care.

Different types of education are needed to support the sustained development of value-based healthcare both nationally and within organizations. E-learning, executive education, implementation support and academic qualifications are all needed. A plurality of high-quality educational offerings is needed around the world in order to grow and sustain the mission. Action learning sets and accredited programmes emphasize practical, collaborative problem solving aligned with value-based healthcare goals.

Patient and public engagement

Patients play a central role in advocating for value-based healthcare by participating in outcome measurement and service design. Public understanding of healthcare challenges is essential for creating external pressure on policymakers to align with value-based healthcare objectives.

Communication

Professionalizing communications is critical to building awareness and credibility for value-based healthcare. Important tools include

- websites, case studies and reports; and

- accessible channels such as webinars and social media, which serve to foster dialogue, problem solving and grass roots engagement.

In my experience, early, informal communication (e.g. Twitter) was instrumental in shaping the value-based healthcare movement and in attracting a diverse network of supporters.

PART II

HOW TO DRIVE VALUE FOR POPULATIONS, PATHWAYS AND PEOPLE

Introduction: a framework for increasing value in healthcare systems

How do we improve outcomes that really matter to people, and how do we contain costs that do not contribute to achieving that outcome? And finally, how do we transform services so that they meet the evolving needs of our populations around the world and mitigate against a burgeoning workforce crisis?

So much needs to be done to create a cultural shift towards value in healthcare and to build the infrastructure to support its implementation that it can be easy to lose sight of why we are doing this in the first place. As we saw in chapter 3, while data is necessary, it is insufficient, on its own, for changing culture and behaviour. We must transform that data into actionable information; we must be clear about all of the interventions in healthcare that improve patient outcomes and reduce costs; and then we must ensure that there are sufficient levers in place to encourage those interventions to take place.

To help structure the thinking around ways to increase value, and manage the complexity that comes with that thinking, I like to think about achieving value in three different ways: value for populations, value across pathways of care, and value for individual people.

Achieving value for the entire population of a country or region requires us to equitably improve outcomes for groups of people with differing needs, regardless of ethnicity, sex, socio-demographic status or healthcare need. Value-based healthcare helps us to address the last item in this list, healthcare need, by segmenting the population into cohorts of people with either a single disease, e.g. lung cancer, or a similar set of needs, e.g. older adults, who may be living with multiple health conditions. Looking at population health also stimulates a broader view of value in health – one that expands outside of healthcare into the community.

There are other applications of value-based healthcare to population health, too. Meeting the totality of population health needs has significant implications for healthcare policy, healthcare system structures and funding, healthcare innovation, and health technology assessment. These issues will be addressed in chapter 6.

Improving outcomes for individual patients requires person-centred care, and we will examine this area in detail in chapter 4.

Chapter 5 will focus on how healthcare providers might increase value (improving outcomes and reducing costs) across pathways of care.

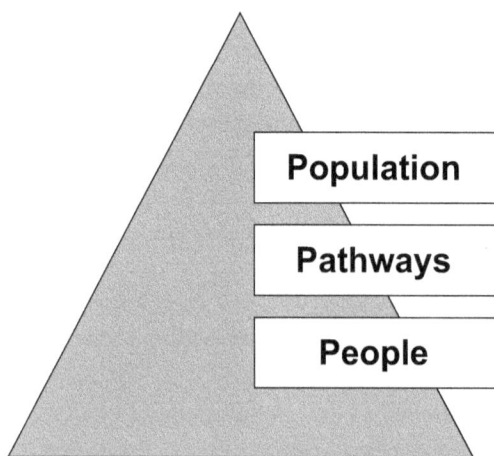

Figure 2. Population, pathways and people.

The value triad: populations, pathways and people

A structured framework helps us to make sense of complexity by focusing on value at three levels.

(1) At the population level
Equitably improve both health outcomes across demographic groups and health needs through segmentation of populations

by conditions (e.g. lung cancer) or needs (e.g. older adults with multimorbidity).

(2) At the pathways level
Providers should collaborate to deliver improved outcomes and reduced costs across care pathways. This is achieved through an analysis of patient needs across the entire pathway of care.

(3) At the people level
Focusing on tailoring care to individual needs and values in the therapeutic consultation.

CHAPTER 4

A person is not a disease: achieving better outcomes for people

'Doctors are men who prescribe medicines of which they know little, to cure diseases of which they know less, in human beings of whom they know nothing.'

— Voltaire

Understanding the value of person-centred care

This chapter is about ascertaining the needs and goals of an individual and then achieving the outcomes that matter to that individual. This process is often referred to as person-centred care.

How may we define person-centred care? The Health Foundation in the United Kingdom has identified four key principles of person-centred care that I think illustrate well why this is a vital part of value-based healthcare.

1. Affording people dignity, compassion and respect.

2. Offering coordinated care, support or treatment.

3. Offering personalized care, support or treatment.

4. Supporting people to recognize and develop their own strengths and abilities to enable them to live an independent and fulfilling life.[1]

There is a lot to unpack in these four principles but it is clear that it will be hard to achieve the best outcomes – and, crucially, outcomes that matter to individuals – without them.

Person-centred care is not to be confused with personalized medicine or precision medicine, which are defined by the Human Genome Project as 'an emerging practice of medicine that uses an individual's genetic profile to guide decisions made in regard to prevention, diagnosis, and treatment of disease'. Personalized medicine will become an increasingly important part of value-based healthcare as we seek to tailor care more specifically to individuals, with the aim of improving outcomes and managing resources more effectively. It is important but not sufficient on its own to deliver person-centredness. We will not be able to achieve this unless we measure standardized outcomes that matter to people. Only then will we be able to start to answer the key question: 'What will happen to somebody *like me* should I take this medicine?' Clinical decision support based on very large outcome datasets should become the norm in this scenario.

In my life as a GP, person-centred care was my bread and butter. I always tried to support my patients, every single day, to achieve the best possible outcomes, and I often engaged in shared decision making to ascertain the best possible course of action to achieve that outcome.[2] British GPs, like many of our generalist counterparts around the world, devote significant time during training to learning consultation skills and different models of the consultation.[3] Historically, one of the other facets of this type of generalism is the notion of 'cradle to grave' care, or continuity. I looked after many of my patients for years, building a trusting relationship over time through multiple contacts with them and their families. Continuity of care, where it can be achieved, has been found to improve patient outcomes, and many of us in the profession are concerned that this aspect is being eroded by a more transactional approach to access to medical appointments.[4]

Tick-box medicine: the downside of formulaic approaches

Over the 24 years of my life as a GP there have been many changes – some good, some not so good. Of those that are not so good, the biggest threat to the philosophy and practice of British generalism are the changes that are pushing us away from relational medicine and towards a more transactional set of interactions with our patients.

The Quality and Outcomes Framework from the new GMS contract in 2003/4 – usually known as the QOF – was the first major change. It was designed to support the embedding of evidence-based medicine in primary care and to reduce unwarranted variation in practice so that we could improve population outcomes.[5]

The upside of QOF was that it incentivized primary care to create chronic disease registers in the electronic record so that we could recall patients for their key tests at appropriate intervals. For example, people living with diabetes need blood tests to monitor the control of their blood glucose and the management of other risk factors such as blood pressure, cholesterol and kidney function. QOF also created incentives for clinical targets against these indicators to be met, with the idea being that this would improve outcomes through reducing unwarranted variation in care.

QOF was highly effective at achieving this aim, but the incentivization framework put two patient groups at a disadvantage. The first group were those for whom the guidelines did not apply, i.e. people that sat outside the 'average'. An example would be frail elderly patients for whom an aggressive blood pressure or blood glucose target might give rise to adverse effects, such as causing them to fall. This is why we need to measure outcomes that matter to people, including their quality of life. The second group were people who, despite multiple contacts from the primary care practice, did not attend or engage with chronic disease management activities. Why was that so? We did not know. The contract allowed primary care to provide an exception report for the patients who did not attend after three interventions, so that the practice was not penalized for the checks not having been done. I believe that this group, often around 10% of the register, were those who were likely to have had worse outcomes. Could we have done more to design care in ways that were more engaging or convenient for them?

One of the unintended consequences of QOF was that it started to create a formulaic and rather mechanistic approach to the care of people with chronic disease, drawing us into a trap of 'tick-box medicine', where the sum of the individual interventions described in the framework was not always greater than the whole. For many patients, we failed to meet their goals and even stopped asking about them in the name of following the evidence-based formula.

The arrival of QOF coincided with a proliferation of single-disease guidelines that started to become tramlines towards an inevitable destination rather than tools to help us navigate the evidence with our patients and achieve their goals. Many people are living with more than one condition, and in a world of increasing sub-specialist expertise, patients need generalists to help view the big picture and integrate all information into better decision making and achieving outcomes that matter. Generalism is about coordination, advocacy and perspective in care. While it does not seek to replace sub-specialist expertise, it is entirely necessary for its success.

The basis of generalism in primary care is relational medicine,[6] and this is our specialism, along with managing undifferentiated illness and a good deal of uncertainty. Given the evolving and complex needs of our population, GPs need to work closely with our generalist cousins in acute medicine and geriatrics if we are to achieve anything that looks at all like integrated medical care for our patients, drawing on the expertise of the specialists of course. For many patients, this type of holistic approach to care will be key to achieving the outcomes that matter to them. It will be just as important as technical brilliance in delivering medical interventions.

People contribute to their own outcomes

People have a profound impact on their own outcomes. They bring their own ideas, beliefs and expectations about health to their consultations, and their actions as a result of their healthcare interactions can either improve or worsen their outcomes, including their quality of life.

The achievement of a positive health outcome is rarely a passive fix administered to a patient by a doctor. Perhaps an antibiotic prescribed for a bacterial infection might fall into this transactional category of medical care, but most interventions require some degree of input by the patient to achieve the optimum outcome. Sometimes this is shorter-term intense activity, such as rehabilitation after surgery, but often it is a lifelong input into managing a chronic condition such as diabetes, rheumatoid arthritis or the after-effects of cancer therapies. Here we see that medicine is an art as well as a science, and part of that art is learning how to support people to work with you to achieve the outcomes that matter to them. This is person-centred care in action, and it needs a relational approach to medical care.

The degree to which people want or can participate in activities to support the best outcome varies enormously, and for many reasons that are nobody's fault. This is why I have always been cautious about signing up to the notion of outcome-based reimbursement systems in healthcare systems. Outcome-based reimbursement rewards or penalizes organizations based on the outcomes they achieve for their patients. Often it is those that are the least able to look after their health that are most disadvantaged in life and who need us the most – people such as Janice, the patient of mine that we met in the book's introduction. We must find the best way to incentivize better outcomes in healthcare, but we must be careful to avoid unintended consequences, e.g. increasing inequalities in healthcare.[7]

People also make different choices about their healthcare. They have differing goals and different preferences for managing their health depending on their environment, family situations or beliefs. These choices often involve trade-offs in outcomes, e.g. a trade-off between *length* of life and *quality* of life. I think back to two of my patients who died of cancer many years ago. They were both women around 50 years old and married with children. Both had been ill, with different types of cancer, for a long time, and they had undergone multiple rounds of gruelling treatment. As their disease progressed to advanced stages and effective treatment options dwindled, they made different decisions about treatment. Sarah, whose children were younger and still at home, decided to try to extend her life by a few extra weeks. She was prepared to accept a reduced quality of life as a result and she endured a heavy symptom burden. Janine chose supportive care alone, preferring to try to achieve quality of life for the short time she had left with her family.

Neither of these decisions was wrong. They were autonomously made. As practitioners, we surely have a duty to support such decisions by providing patients with as much information as possible on the likely impact of their decisions. The only way we can do that is if we are routinely embedding outcomes measurement (clinical and patient-reported) in care and building large databases of what actually happens to patients in real-life treatment scenarios – the ultimate goal of real-world evidence.[8] This forms the basis of learning health and care systems and, later, of value-based procurement of technologies in medicine, where reimbursement is linked to real patient outcomes.

Sometimes clinical guidelines and our internal biases cause us to make assumptions about the treatment choices of our patients. This can result in undertreatment too. A patient of mine, James, was in his mid-seventies and had developed atrial fibrillation, a common disorder as we age. Atrial fibrillation causes an irregular heartbeat that increases the likelihood of developing blood clots leading to stroke. The irregular rhythm may also be much faster than normal and put a strain on the heart. Treatments are focused on preventing clots (anti-coagulant medication) and either controlling the rate (medication) or correcting the rhythm (cardioversion or cardiac ablation). An excellent description and treatment decision aid has been produced by the National Institute for Health and Care Excellence (NICE) in the United Kingdom.[9]

The problem for James was that in terms of physical performance, he was not an 'average' man. He was a lifelong athlete and still trained daily as well as participating in half marathons and hill walking. As a result, his normal resting heart rate had been around 50 beats per minute before he developed atrial fibrillation. At diagnosis, his resting heart rate was 110 beats per minute. Initial therapeutic intervention with medication reduced his heart rate to around 90 beats per minute. For some people this might have been tolerable, but for James it meant that he was symptomatic as it was still way higher than his baseline. Even worse, the medication made him tired and he was unable to exercise in the way he had done all his life. This was having a significant impact on his quality of life, particularly with respect to his mental health and wellbeing.

The NICE decision aid referenced above does not cover this eventuality. James's medical team needed to help James reach a decision about the treatment option that would control his atrial fibrillation and prevent stroke while also returning his functioning to the maximum realistic level possible. This is the art of medicine. We must always remember that we are caring for a person, not a disease.

How PROMs can support person-centred care

Over the last ten years of PROMs implementation across multiple clinical settings and clinical conditions, the Value in Health team and the clinical teams across Wales saw first hand the beneficial impact of PROMs as a tool to support person-centred care. The first thing they observed was how the use of PROMs could alter the dynamics of a therapeutic consultation, including reversing the power dynamics between clinician and patient.[10]

In the Parkinson's disease clinic in the Aneurin Bevan University Health Board, patients and their carers were asked to complete a PROM on arrival at clinic and immediately prior to the consultation. This simple intervention enabled them to flag what was most bothering them that day and put them in a position to lead and prioritize the discussion. It was very powerful. Patients and carers also began to discuss their disease with each other as they completed the PROM, creating impromptu peer support in the waiting room. Later, patients told us how much they valued this interaction.

We quickly realized that PROMs implementation was not merely a data collection exercise on which to perform future analyses: it was also a valuable structured communication between patient and clinician. In the context of a chronic illness, it was a milestone in a person's life and a detailed assessment of symptom burden, and as such it was more than just an evaluation of the success or failure of a treatment. If this structured assessment was done in the right way and was embraced by both parties, it was very effective in supporting person-centred care. Viewing PROMs as a tool for supporting care (such as a blood test or a physical examination) seemed very important, but a cultural shift for clinicians and patients was required if doing so was to become mainstream.

Using PROMs in the consultation also started to raise health literacy among patients and carers attending clinic. Patients told us that this was because the completing of the PROM promoted open discussion about symptoms that may have previously been difficult to talk about, such as disinhibition or compulsive behaviour as one of the side effects of anti-Parkinsonian medication.[11] Additionally, people were sometimes made aware during this process of symptoms that they had not linked to their Parkinson's disease.

We saw, therefore, that PROMs data alongside the articulation of individual goals and preferences for care was the optimum approach to encouraging person-centred care. We observed this phenomenon time and again with other conditions too. Imagine how this approach could have helped James, Sarah and Janine.

Using PROMs to tailor access to care and support new care models

As we matured in our approach to the digital deployment of PROMs in direct care of patients, we uncovered another way in which they supported person-centred care. This happened in the inflammatory bowel disease (IBD) clinic, and it enabled flexible access to clinical support for this patient population.

IBD is a debilitating chronic condition that can cause abdominal pain and multiple episodes of bloody diarrhoea each day. If untreated it can progress to serious and sometimes life-threatening complications. The population affected by this disease tend to be younger and of working age, often with young families. Modern drugs have revolutionized the care of people with IBD, and most patients enjoy much better clinical outcomes and quality of life as a result. They do, however, require regular blood test monitoring to avoid serious adverse effects. Patients with IBD told us that when they were well and their condition was stable, they did not want to visit the hospital for routine follow-ups as this did not add any value for them. Conversely, if they had a flare-up of the disease, they wanted to be seen as quickly as possible for emergency treatment. This was essential if they were to avoid complications and get back to normal life as quickly as possible.

As well as flexible models of access to care, people wanted access to their disease and medication monitoring blood test results and other information about their health so that they could be proactive in self-management. This access to information digitally is one important element of supporting self-management in the modern medical age – it is a key principle of person-centred care. As we develop value-based models of care, consideration should be given to strategies for systematically investing in supported self-management. This will be critical to supporting the achievement of good outcomes in the growing population of people in society living with at least one chronic disease. Supported self-management does not happen by accident or by magic. It should be considered as much an intervention in the pathway of care as a medicine, surgery or other procedure.

Coming back to the example of our IBD clinic, we saw the team work with patients to devise a flexible access model in the clinic. In this model, patients who wanted to be seen could trigger a PROM assessment so that the team could instantly see the severity of the individual's symptom burden and prioritize their appointment accordingly. Similarly, stable patients could be monitored remotely, supported by PROM assessment alongside their monitoring blood tests. This enabled those patients to avoid unwanted and unnecessary appointments, releasing capacity in clinical time and decreasing the burden of care processes for patients. Additionally, the team were able to prioritize the most vulnerable patients in clinic: those who were unable to complete a PROM remotely.

Boosting self-management

A good example of where patients' involvement in their own care is essential for improving outcomes occurs in musculoskeletal disease. As our societies age, the numbers of us with osteoarthritis are rising. Total knee and hip replacement surgery has changed the lives of many people living with this condition. However, these surgeries are not a passive fix, and neither are they without risk. We know that tailored exercise and weight management programmes can reduce painful symptoms, delaying the need for surgery. Even more importantly, we know that people who have managed their weight and have engaged in exercise prior to surgery tend to have fewer complications and better outcomes from the intervention. Programmes to support people to manage this condition are therefore very important. One such programme has been in operation in Swansea Bay, West Wales, since 2021.

Under the leadership of head physiotherapist Chris Lambert, an exercise and lifestyle (ELP) programme was introduced in 2021, supported by the health board's value-based healthcare team. It combined exercise, education and weight management into a single service. Patients directly referred from primary care with a suspected osteoarthritis diagnosis were able to access specialist assessment and investigations, combined with lifestyle management delivered as a supervised community-based programme. Self-management options were available for those unable to commit to the supervised programme, and these have been shown to be equally effective.

Patient outcomes captured in clinic or remotely via a digital platform demonstrated an average improvement in Oxford knee score of 2.5. This represented a significant improvement in the patient-reported outcome measure favoured by British orthopaedic surgeons. A weight reduction of 3.6 kilograms and a reduction in secondary care orthopaedic referrals by 17% were also seen.

The service has maintained its excellent outcomes and has since expanded to include hip osteoarthritis patients in 2023. The ELP programme continues to evolve and is now using patient goals to enable a patient-centred care approach. At present, the service manages up to 1,250 patients per year, but it has plans to expand its education and self-management offer via a new front-end patient group workshop. Successful roll-out of the workshops could allow an increase of up to 50% in yearly osteoarthritis referrals to access the programme, through remodelling and better use of existing resources. The group workshops also allow for peer support networks to become established – an important factor in building health in local communities.

Giving people access to their information: the key to coordinated care and self-management

At the beginning of the chapter I included a four-part definition of person-centred healthcare provided by the Health Foundation. I now want to come back to the second and third parts of that definition: 'coordinated care, support or treatment'; and 'supporting people to recognise and develop their own strengths and abilities to enable them to live an independent and fulfilling life'. There is a driver of both of these goals that is key to their achievement: patient access to their own health data.

The stories in this chapter have shown how important it is for care and clinical guidelines to be personalized and tailored to individuals if we are to achieve the outcomes that matter to them. What about the other three prerequisites for person-centred care that appear on the Health Foundation list?

Let us tackle coordinated care first. When one speaks to patients, it is rarely long before you hear frustrating experiences about how disjointed their care has been. Tales abound of how they have had to repeat their story multiple times to different professionals involved in their care; about delays in being able to access their results and other information; about multiple unnecessary 'in person' attendances at clinics and hospitals; and about not being able to access care when they needed it. These occurrences are not simply a minor annoyance: they cost patients time and money, and in the case of missing information, they can have a detrimental effect on patient safety. They represent system failure and are a major cause of waste.[*] In short, just about everywhere in the world, most patients would agree that we are not good at coordinating their care and we are not good at integrating their care across different healthcare providers, who often do not adequately share data to support that integration and coordination. The only reliable way to achieve this is for patients to have the power to see and control their own health information, both sharing and prohibiting access where appropriate (and alerting us to mistakes – a critical safety component to all this).

It is encouraging, therefore, to see that governments around the world are committing to people's right to access their data. For example, in 2021 the G7 countries agreed five principles and ambitions regarding patient access to their health data:

- online access to records;
- use of own information to manage patient health;
- patients contributing to their health record;
- offering online access to health information by healthcare providers; and
- an audit trail of who has accessed a patient's record.

Countries are doing this at their own pace, bound by their own laws and healthcare systems. However, encouraging progress is being seen, with Estonia providing a particularly excellent example.

---

[*] Waste in healthcare (not a popular term) is anything that does not contribute to the desired patient outcome in the most efficient way.

Integrated care and value-based healthcare are intrinsic to each other. We will come back to integrated care delivery later, in the book's final chapter.

If people are to be able to get the most out of their interaction with healthcare professionals and to be able to stay healthy and/or to manage chronic conditions such as diabetes, heart failure and asthma, they need more than just access to data: that data needs to be turned into information that is relatable, understandable and can be acted upon. This sounds very simple, but it takes a great deal of thoughtful work to pick it all apart and deliver on it. Information must take many different forms if it is to be impactful for different groupings dependent on age, culture, gender, levels of health literacy, and so on. Self-management also takes a lot of confidence, and confidence can only be built – it does not magically appear. People therefore need coaching, and they need flexible access to their clinical team for advice.

One size does not fit all: embedding these lessons in healthcare

Raising health literacy and supporting patients with access to their health information to help them manage their condition is a major pillar in improving the outcomes that matter – and, therefore, of reducing the vast costs of acute healthcare utilization (emergency department attendances for disease exacerbations, longer lengths of stay in hospital, interventions to address organ damage, and so on) that result from suboptimal disease management and preventable poor outcomes. Patients live with their conditions 365 days a year. This sounds obvious, but it makes sense to understand how to support them more fully in playing their part in achieving a good outcome. In general, we do not do this well or invest nearly enough time and other resources in improvement. When it comes to supporting patients, one size does not fit all – we need an understanding of patient activation[12] if we are to meet everyone's needs effectively.

Patient activation describes the knowledge, skills and confidence a person has in managing their own health and care, and it is an important consideration when designing tailored and effective services to support people living with chronic illness. Payers and providers in healthcare have a responsibility to invest significantly in activities that support patients in managing their health at home. It is the right thing to do for people and it will improve their outcomes, and it is also of major importance if we are to achieve healthcare system sustainability and equity of access to healthcare into the future.

I was interested to see that some of the greatest initial benefits of implementing PROMs in care were to be found not in comparing results, but in improving the person-centredness of care. This is of course good news if we are to achieve the high response rates for PROM assessments that are needed to create robust and inclusive datasets for analysis. For example, in evaluating real-world effectiveness of new medical technologies, Santeon, a Dutch hospital group, are leading the way with their value-based research programme in this field. In the Dutch healthcare context, value-based healthcare implementation has maintained a strong focus on shared decision making. Santeon is using its outcome data to create decision aids for patients to help them make decisions about their care based on likely outcomes 'for somebody like me'. The seven-hospital network has harmonized its data onto a single platform, enabling tools to be created to support person-centred care. In kidney care, for example, they say this:

> For a patient with kidney failure, for example, we have created dashboards to explore the different treatment options available at different stages of the condition. These provide insights to help clinicians in determining the best treatment for care – for example, at what stage a transplant, dialysis, or food intervention is most appropriate.

The Santeon team, including Willem Jan Bos, Pieter de Bey and Paul Van der Naat, have been true pioneers of this approach, as has Linetta Koppert at Erasmus Medical Centre.

I am sure that by now you can appreciate the perversity of healthcare reimbursement models that pay for activity such as a clinic visit without tying that visit to outcome in some way. These reimbursement models are actively counterproductive, not only to patient experience of care and care burden, but also to the effective use of staffing resources in healthcare systems. This is also true, to an extent, of activity-based performance targets in public health systems that are not fee for service, such as that in Wales. We should be designing reimbursement and other incentives that encourage the development and adoption of innovative person-centred care models in our healthcare systems. Care models that are flexible and that are co-designed with patients to meet their needs, focusing on outcome not attendance at a healthcare facility. Self-management and person-centred care do not happen by magic: they are interventions as important as surgery or medicines, and they need both our attention and investment in resources.

Key lessons from chapter 4

Challenges of formulaic approaches in healthcare

Tick-box medicine
Frameworks such as QOF, while designed to improve outcomes, risk reducing care to formulaic processes, neglecting individual goals.

Multimorbidity management
Sub-specialization and single-disease guidelines can fail to address the complexity of patients with multiple chronic

conditions. Generalists are critical in coordinating care and integrating various inputs to achieve holistic outcomes, which should be measured.

The art of medicine: relational and holistic care

Relational medicine
Building long-term, trusting relationships between clinicians and patients improves outcomes and patient satisfaction. Continuity of care is critical for achieving this – a point highlighted in the PROMs and PREMs (patient-reported experience measures) captured in the OECD PaRIS survey.

Holistic view
Outcomes depend on viewing patients as whole people, not diseases. This involves accounting for individual preferences, trade-offs (e.g. length of life versus quality of life), co-morbidities and life circumstances.

Role of PROMs

Enhancing consultations
PROMs shift the dynamic of consultations, allowing patients to highlight their priorities and empowering them to lead discussions.

Supporting health literacy
PROMs encourage open communication, making patients more aware of their symptoms and conditions.

Tailored models of care
PROMs enable flexible care pathway design, reducing unnecessary appointments and optimizing treatment choices while prioritizing urgent care needs.

Broader impact
Beyond data collection, PROMs serve as tools to support person-centred care and to create datasets for real-world evidence.

Supporting self-management and patient activation

Self-management as an intervention
Effective chronic disease management depends on empowering patients with tools, information and support to manage their health outside of clinical settings. Getting this right is critical to achieving a good outcome.

Tailored approaches
One-size-fits-all models are inadequate; understanding patient activation levels is key to customizing effective support for people.

Digital tools
Providing patients with access to health data (e.g. blood test results) helps them proactively manage their conditions, improves health literacy and avoids preventable complications.

Trade-offs and patient autonomy in decision making

Individual preferences
Patients make different trade-offs based on their values (see the example earlier of Sarah and Janine choosing life extension versus quality of life). Clinicians must respect these choices by providing clear information about likely outcomes.

Avoiding bias
Healthcare providers must avoid making assumptions about patient preferences, which can lead to undertreatment or overtreatment.

The role of real-world evidence

Outcome measurement
Embedding outcomes measurement (both clinical and patient-reported) into care supports informed decision making and continuous learning. When we have acquired large outcome datasets (real-world data) we will be able to help patients understand the outcomes that they as individuals can expect, whatever healthcare option they opt for.

Future directions
Real-world evidence can guide the value-based procurement of technologies, aligning reimbursement with real-life patient outcomes.

CHAPTER 5

Making a difference: driving value aross pathways of care

'However beautiful the strategy, you should occasionally look at the results.'

— Winston Churchill

Understanding value in pathways of care

One of the most important principles of value-based healthcare in any context is the need to organize care around the needs of the patient in a way that is integrated and appears seamless to the person receiving that care. In the last chapter I focused on the importance of person-centred care and on how we could increase value for individual patients and healthcare practitioners or services. Now I will turn to a greater challenge: how to achieve high-value care (improved outcomes and reduced costs) across pathways of care. This requires care integration, often across several care settings.

Whole pathways of care encapsulate prevention, timely diagnosis, optimized intervention, follow-up care and palliative care (see figure 3). It follows that the highest-value activities from a healthcare system sustainability perspective fall earlier in the pathway: in the prevention and early diagnosis space. This is because preventing a disease or curing one are the best outcomes of all. It is ironic, then, that this section of the pathway is one that is frequently neglected and not optimized, even though it is relatively inexpensive to put that right. Within healthcare systems, we often tend to 'default to rescue'. That is where we focus our resources, and this is, in part, why we are now in crisis.

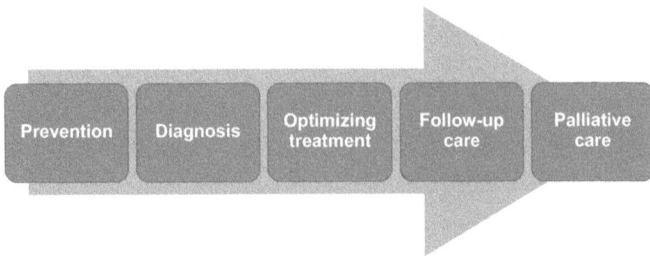

Figure 3. A generic whole pathway of care.

The generic pathway of care for those with a health condition such as type 2 diabetes or lung cancer, or for a cohort of people with similar needs (e.g. older adults), includes the entire continuum of care from prevention through to end-of-life care (where applicable).

To achieve maximum value for a patient or a population we must look at the outcomes we are achieving and the costs of all the activities and interventions involved in achieving those outcomes across the whole pathway. We can then take a view about what we need to do to improve both those outcomes and the sustainability of the healthcare system, supported by the judicious use of incentives. We can see that if we focus on existing service provision, e.g. hospital care, we might miss how we could improve value for patients across the whole pathway as well as missing the opportunity for care innovations. This is especially true when we think about moving care closer to home and supporting self-management.

This approach helps us to ensure that we are maximizing all the highest-value interventions. In the case of lung cancer, this means paying as much attention to smoking cessation and early diagnosis as it does to treating people with the latest chemotherapeutic discovery. Here we see an overlap between population and pathway value. The difficulty for many countries and providers is that care is usually fragmented in some way. This could be external fragmentation, with the total pathway of care being spread across several organizations, or it could be that care is internally disjointed, e.g. across a number of departments in a hospital. Given the multifaceted nature of value-based healthcare implementation, we found that a pragmatic approach was needed. The ideal is to understand costs and outcomes and integrate care across the whole pathway. However, when starting out, most organizations will not be able to do that, so doing what we can with the segments of pathway within our own organization is a reasonable place to begin. Note, though, that there is a risk in this approach that we create further distance between hospital and primary care.

Now let us consider a common misstep in driving value in pathway care: seeing it as quality improvement alone.

Quality alone is not value

The Institute for Healthcare Improvement defines quality improvement (QI) as a systematic approach to solving problems and improving care. QI methodologies provide an important mindset and toolbox with which to improve care processes and make care effective and safe. QI is, therefore, an essential component of value-based care.

The World Health Organization defines quality care as that which is effective (evidence based), safe (without harm) and person centred (responsive to individual preference and need). Often, QI initiatives focus on care process improvement, such as increased compliance to clinical guidelines, with the aim of improving safety, outcome or efficiency. Unfortunately, compliance with clinical guidelines and processes does not always guarantee high-value care. This is not meant to be a criticism of QI: we need process improvement in services to help us manage resources and improve patient care. Quality care may increase the likelihood of a good outcome, but it does not make one inevitable, and unless we measure patient outcomes we cannot assume that it has worked. Let us look at diabetes management as an illustration of this.

There is strong evidence that people living with diabetes should have regular checks on eight key parameters, often referred to as the 'bundle of eight' care processes. In the United Kingdom these are almost always carried out in primary care (see table 1). An important hospital-based ninth process is eye screening. The purpose of these checks is to assess the degree to which a person's diabetes and the associated risk factors are tightly controlled, as we know that, in general, tight control improves outcomes by reducing the likelihood of major complications in diabetes (i.e. cardiovascular events, amputation, sight loss and kidney failure requiring dialysis).

Table 1. Evidence-based care processes to support good outcomes in diabetes.

	Test	Rationale
1	HbA1C	To assess diabetes control in recent months
2	Blood pressure	A significant cardiovascular risk factor
3	Serum creatinine	A measure of kidney function
4	Urine albumin/creatinine ratio	Helps identify kidney disease early
5	Serum cholesterol	A risk factor for cardiovascular disease
6	Foot check (pulse and sensation)	Important for assessing risk of tissue damage in the extremities to prevent ulceration and, ultimately, amputation
7	Body mass index	A risk factor for cardiovascular and other diseases
8	Smoking history	A cardiovascular risk factor
9	Digital eye screening	To identify and treat diabetic eye disease early

The application of QI methodology to variation in uptake of these checks improves adherence to the guidelines and might result in an alteration of treatment with the aim of improving the outcome. For some patients, this could result in an improvement in their blood pressure or in blood test results, but for others it might not. Chronic diabetes management requires a good deal of input from the patient to achieve a good outcome – from tight control of diet to taking care of one's feet and monitoring blood glucose levels. Supported self-management therefore becomes an important intervention, and one that is often overlooked. We need to understand patient-reported outcomes in addition to clinical outcomes to appreciate this nuance and to adjust the services provided accordingly. Excellent outcomes are a product of teamwork between patients and clinicians!

Using patient-reported data to support service redesign

As we saw in chapter 4, if we are to transform services for value, we must gain a better understanding of what people need to help them manage their chronic conditions in their everyday lives, away from formal healthcare. Fortunately, there are good ways of doing this.

For example, the P3CEQ tool is an 11-item patient questionnaire that measures people's experience of goal setting, empowerment/activation, confidence in self-management, carer involvement, care planning, decision making, information and communication. The tool was deployed as part of the OECD PaRIS survey, a groundbreaking international survey of patient-reported experiences and outcomes in those living with a chronic disease. The survey's first set of results was published in February 2025.[1] The P3CEQ tool comes with a commissioner's guide on how to develop services that enable far more patient engagement and therefore better outcomes and reduced costs. Self-management does not happen by magic!

Another example of this type of tool is the Diabetes Distress Q, which forms part of the ICHOM standard set of outcome measures for diabetes.[2,3] This focuses on the psychological impact of diabetes, confidence in managing the disease, and the quality of interaction with the medical team. Driving value-based healthcare impact requires a collaborative effort to respond to datasets such as these. Our patients are telling us what they need first hand. We ignore that information at our peril.

Some years ago, I talked to Rose, an inspirational health psychologist, who was working with teenagers living with type 1 diabetes. The transition from childhood to adulthood can be a particularly difficult time, and without expert psychology input, diabetes control can be quite unstable, leading to adverse outcomes such as diabetic ketoacidosis, a life-threatening emergency. Rose had demonstrated that this group of people had much better outcomes if they were given dedicated psychological support, and she had reduced the rate of diabetic ketoacidosis within her organization by a highly significant amount. Services such as Rose's should be given equal importance to drugs and surgeries if we are to achieve the best outcomes for our patients and for the population.

In summary, data such as this might reveal why some patients are struggling to do well and might hint at what is missing, thereby allowing us to redesign care to better support those patients. By focusing on patient outcomes resulting from the entire pathway of care, value-based healthcare therefore adds a further dimension, by prompting us to look at the gaps. What are we missing that is needed to improve the outcome for the patient and to reduce costs?

So, quality and value are intrinsically linked, but distinct.

Why is this distinction important?

Making a distinction between quality and value might seem like unnecessary academic navel-gazing, but I discovered the hard way that it was of practical relevance. In the early days of introducing value-based healthcare, I encountered opposition – even hostility – from some involved with quality improvement and Prudent Healthcare. I am not sure why this was. In my view, all of these movements and methodologies are tools in the box towards a common aim: better outcomes for people and sustainable healthcare systems. I have always believed that the disciplines of quality improvement and value-based healthcare are intimately linked and require each other. Value-based healthcare is a data-driven delivery mechanism for Prudent Healthcare and its like abroad, so teams working in these fields need to work together, not compete with each other.

During the early days of Prudent Healthcare, projects were typically assigned to a separate workstream in organizational strategy with a cost improvement target approach. There was an assumption that it was up to the clinical teams to reduce unwarranted variation through quality improvement methods to the extent that financial savings would be made. In other healthcare systems where activity generates a fee, I am certain this manifests as an expectation for clinical teams to increase productivity to increase revenue for a hospital. Context matters, but drivers of human behaviour are generally the same everywhere. Not only is this disengaging for clinicians, but it misses the point. Being 'prudent' should have been everybody's business managerially, clinically and financially. It should have been a golden seam that ran through everything we did. With its focus on outcomes and costs together, value-based healthcare forces everyone to take responsibility.

Now let us look at some of the key approaches to increasing value across pathways of care.

Increasing value across pathways of care

There are myriad ways to improve outcomes and reduce costs across pathways of care, and the focus of how to do that will be influenced both by the context and structure of a country's healthcare system and by the patient group concerned.

Optimizing intervention and tailoring care to patient cohorts

People's needs are rarely uniform, even if they are living with the same disease. Yet all too often we adopt a one-size-fits-all service for all patients, resulting in no one's needs being entirely met and creating an unsatisfactory experience for both patients and their carers. Outpatient clinics are a classic example of this, as we saw in the Parkinson's disease clinic described in earlier chapters. A one-size-fits-all approach also tends to be resource intensive, particularly in relation to clinical time as caseloads grow.

It is very important to identify these cohorts of patients so that their unmet needs can be characterized, quantified and costed. The cost of not meeting need and the cost of adverse patient events is a very important calculation to make. The cost of poor outcomes forms the basis of an argument for changing funding flows to deliver care in a way that better meets the needs of a given cohort. Outcome data, including patient-reported outcomes, can inform how we might improve on decision making with respect to resource allocation as it comprises a needs assessment.

For example, in our early work on Parkinson's disease, the outcome data highlighted that there were three distinct cohorts of patients coming to clinic with differing needs yet being treated with a one-size-fits-all approach to care. Taking this approach meant that there was suboptimal treatment for every group, leading to an inability to drive better outcomes and improve experience of care despite the best attempts of the clinical team.

The data showed that newly diagnosed patients had a burden of psychological morbidity and needed more support for their mental health and wellbeing. Patients with advanced disease and multiple complex symptomatology needed to see numerous different healthcare professionals – physiotherapists, speech therapists, neurologists, clinical nurse specialists

– but this was not coordinated well. This meant that these patients had even more frequent and disjointed attendances, and that was also consuming more resources. It was possible to make the case for an integrated approach to care. Meanwhile, patients with stable disease perhaps did not always need as many appointments, but they did need the comfort of flexible access to the clinical team when they needed it. Costing and outcome data together can better inform effective resource allocation to meet people's needs.

The impact of growing caseload, which is inevitable as more and more people live with chronic disease, is profound. Pressure on clinical time as more patients need to be seen in an old outpatient model of care begins to cause burnout in healthcare professionals, contributing further to the workforce crisis. We saw another example of this at the Aneurin Bevan University Health Board in a team led by the head clinical nurse specialist in heart failure, Linda Edmunds. Again, the vast caseload of patients was making things difficult for patients and staff. Growing the service was challenging due to financial constraints and unavailability of qualified personnel, so Linda knew that they had to do something different. She and her team introduced measurement of the ICHOM standard set of outcomes for heart failure into the heart failure clinics.

As with the Parkinson's disease example, three distinct groups of patients emerged: newly diagnosed patients; a group of patients with stable disease (as indicated by the clinical and patient-reported outcomes); and a group with severe disease and complex health and social care needs. Having the outcome data at their fingertips gave the team and their patients the opportunity to develop a new model of care. To increase capacity in the clinic, stable patients were discharged to the care of their primary care physician with a quick route back into clinic in case of need. New patients had a dedicated service. They were seen rapidly and had a coordinated approach to optimizing their medication. This meant that they were on the required doses of heart failure drugs within three months, something that was not reliably happening prior to the change. In turn, this improved patient outcomes and significantly reduced the number of hospital readmissions with heart failure. Meanwhile, people with severe, advanced disease were now receiving a person-centred and tailored approach to care that helped to prevent crises and enabled patients to receive palliative care at the right time and to be cared for appropriately at home.

This is value-based service remodelling in action. Needs-led, and supported by patient outcome data at every step. For this to happen, PROMs must be embedded in direct care and it needs to be visible to the clinician and, ideally, the patient. We uncovered some useful principles for embedding PROMs for use in the consultation. First, the PROM should be imported from patient-facing software and incorporated into the electronic health record such that it can easily be accessed with a simple mouse click. Second, clinicians wanted a more detailed breakdown of the PROM score, i.e. drilling down into individual symptoms and their trends. We designed this functionality as a simple click on the aggregate score. To make it easier for the information to be assimilated quickly, scores were also colour coded from red to amber to green, representing a spectrum of severity of symptoms from severe to absent.

Reducing low-value care; adopting high-value care

Low-value care is inherently wasteful: it does not contribute to an improved outcome for a person and therefore unnecessarily consumes resources.

Patients are quickly able to identify many examples of low-value care: a procedure that did not make them better, for example, or a drug that gave them side effects or an appointment they did not need. Healthcare professionals might well be able to come up with a few more: a blood test or scan that has been ordered but that is not going to change management, for example, or procedures without a convincing evidence base for effectiveness.

Over the years, we did a lot of work trying to reduce low-value prescribing and scans and to minimize unnecessary referrals to specialists through the development of clinical pathway guidelines. This has also been the goal of global movements such as Choosing Wisely International, who have carried out a lot of patient engagement on this topic.

I also persuaded the Welsh government to refresh its policy position on low-value procedures so that we could track activity against interventions for which the evidence base was poor. This resulted in the creation of a National Clinical Effectiveness Group comprising clinicians, experts in health technology assessment and representatives from the health board. The group's task was to develop a consensus for a list of 'interventions not normally undertaken' that would then be tracked and reduced. It is interesting to see other countries – notably the Singapore Ministry of Health – begin to align the related disciplines of value-based healthcare and health technology assessment.[4]

Reducing low-value care is clearly worthwhile – and as healthcare professionals we do have a responsibility for some stewardship here – but there was nothing more annoying to me as a doctor than being required to save organizational resources while simultaneously observing a lack of attention given to the adoption of high-value interventions. That had to change in my view, so I wrote into the terms of reference that the group would ultimately also have a responsibility to track the adoption and implementation of new technologies of very high value to patients.

A good example of this is flash glucose monitoring, which uses modern sensors that allow people with diabetes to regularly track their blood glucose throughout the day without the need for painful finger prick testing. This makes a massive difference to people's confidence, to their ability to manage their diabetes, and ultimately to their outcomes. Have you ever tried pricking your finger with a lancet for a point-of-care test? I have. It hurts, and I would not want to do it several times a day, every day.

Driving improvement in Wales: prioritization and focus

Despite making a lot of progress in obtaining and curating outcome and other datasets to support value-based improvement in Wales, I was disappointed that there was still a lack of national, systemic focus on this data. It was even more frustrating because of the myriad of local organizational value-based healthcare projects that were now bearing fruit.

There were a few reasons for the lack of systemic focus. Partly, despite discussion of value-based care now being quite common across the Welsh health system, I think custom and practice kept people focused on activity and finance data. This issue was not helped by a lack of clear prioritization for what issues to tackle first and where we most needed to improve nationally. When everything is prioritized, nothing is prioritized.

Fortunately, a high-profile board was convened, chaired by the director general of the NHS in Wales. The board was called the Value and Sustainability Board, and while a lot of its work was just about improving operational grip on service management, it had a workstream dedicated to value-based service improvements. I decided to use this to try to create focus around some limited priorities for value-based healthcare at a national level. I started by asking national clinical directors in diabetes, frailty, cardiology and orthopaedics what they felt their top three priority interventions would be if we were to make the biggest difference to outcomes in diabetes, osteoporosis (and fragility fractures), heart failure and hip and knee arthroplasty. Figure 4 demonstrates what this looked like for diabetes (prevention applying to type 2 diabetes).

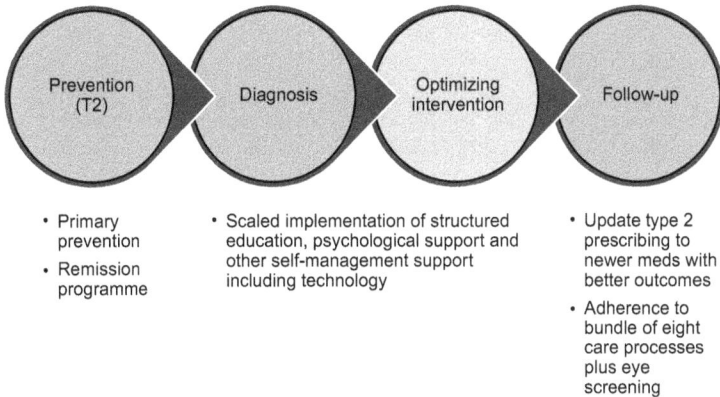

Figure 4. Priority interventions in diabetes.

You will notice in the figure the healthy mix of prevention, person-centred care and adoption of high-value care; the work brought together a powerful coalition from the national diabetes network, Public Health Wales (the national public health organization) and the Welsh Value in Health Centre.

High-value care meant not just technology adoption but also doing the basics of care well. The idea was to get the Value and Sustainability Board to track these interventions with strong evidence bases for driving better outcomes and reduced costs, alongside outcome and costing data that was already present in the national diabetes dashboard.

The approach got traction immediately, and the intention was to spread the initiative to other clinical pathways, backed up by the data-visualization techniques my team had learned at Scuola Superiore Sant'Anna in Pisa. I received some criticism initially for taking this approach from those who thought it was a little reductionist and was potentially excluding other important areas of work. I was very clear that this was not meant to be exclusive. People could improve outcomes wherever they saw fit, but the intention was to create focus, drive and action around improving outcomes in areas where there were important systemic issues and where there was excellent clinical leadership.

The thorny issue of prevention

One of the other interventions we have struggled to fully address in Wales is the prevention agenda – something all countries must focus on if we are going to build healthier communities and reduce healthcare costs.

In Wales, the problem is not our approach to public health. We have excellent public health policy, professionals and practice in our little country. The problem is not our healthcare structures either. We have a system that arguably lends itself to delivering value-based healthcare more than many others, because each of the integrated health boards in Wales has oversight of healthcare paths end to end: from prevention to palliative care. In our capitation-based payment system we have the ability, at least in theory, to move resources across pathways to maximize high-value activity, including prevention. The trouble is that the system is under pressure and is being given other, more immediate targets to focus on. For every service business case put to the health boards, a short-term return on investment is expected – something that prevention struggles to demonstrate. We all say we want more prevention, and then we fail to work towards it.

One of the tactics we championed at the Welsh Value in Health Centre was a drive towards maximizing the impact of secondary prevention in chronic disease because of the shorter-term measurable impact on outcomes. Secondary prevention aims to minimize the impact and the adverse consequences of a chronic disease, and there are diverse programmes of work taking place across Wales in diabetes, alcohol harm reduction and cardiopulmonary disease.

Adapting value-based healthcare to pathways of care globally

As we seek to improve outcomes worldwide, we come across many contexts in which it is neither feasible nor practical to measure a comprehensive set of outcome data, such as that proposed by ICHOM. But this does not matter. It is still possible to make inroads into improving outcomes and overall value once we have identified a need for a particular patient group.

In Sub-Saharan Africa, for instance, universal access to healthcare remains a major challenge. Pharmaccess was founded in 2001 by Professor Joep Lange to find innovative solutions to making antiretroviral drugs available to patients in Sub-Saharan Africa through public–private partnerships. The rapid rise of mobile technology has enabled Pharmaccess to accelerate the journey towards making health markets work to achieve universal coverage. The company typically uses mobile technology to monitor healthcare utilization (e.g. clinic visits and associated costs) and simple outcome data points to evidence value creation.

Some years ago, Pharmaccess created a value-based healthcare programme called MomCare, which was designed to support Kenyan women throughout their pregnancy and on into the postpartum period, improving outcomes for mothers and their babies. The model of care is completely funded by social donors via Pharmaccess.[5] Patients, providers and the payer are connected by mobile technology, and there is total transparency around basic outcome data and costs. MomCare identified significant mental health problems within this population of pregnant women and wanted to design an intervention to support them, but there was a problem. There were a very large number of women needing help and huge gaps in the primary care workforce available. A creative approach was needed.

This is what happened. At the booking appointment, women were screened with a simple two-question depression PROM: the PHQ-2. Those with a positive screen went on to have more detailed assessments using the PHQ-9 and the Edinburgh Post-natal Depression Score (EDPS). Only severely affected women required onward specialist referral. The remainder were supported by a novel service in the community, co-designed with local women to ensure that it was culturally appropriate.

The gaps in the primary care workforce were addressed by recruiting a network of professionally supported community health workers and through a group therapy model. This was all hugely successful. The key point here was the light-touch outcomes measurement used as both a needs assessment and a service-effectiveness assessment. This enabled confidence to be built that the innovative service model was sustainable and effective. It also made very good use of local resources.

Finally, attention to meaningful co-design of the innovative model (think back to the Prudent Healthcare example in chapter 1) meant that the service was extremely well received and well attended by the women who needed it. This Kenyan case study is a good illustration of why quality and value in healthcare are not the same. Quality improvement of existing services would not have met the need here. The problem needed an entirely novel approach – one enabled by outcomes measurement.

Another challenging scenario is presented by extremes of geography. Northwestern Queensland in Australia presents us with a good example of this issue. The Primary Health Network there is using value-based healthcare as the basis for its Healthy Outback Communities strategy.[6] Recognizing difficulties relating to accessing care and the fragmentation of services, the emphasis here is on forming an alliance of providers who are focused on achieving outcomes. The intention is to move away from individual providers measuring their own input through counting activity alone, and instead shift towards collective

responsibility for measuring and improving outcomes – particularly those relating to the life course and to the prevention and
management of chronic disease. As in Kenya, emphasis is placed
on co-designing care in a way that is culturally sensitive. The
team's aspiration is to move towards the ICHOM standard set
of outcome measures for adults and children, but the key ingre-
dient here is again to focus on healthcare provider partnerships
and relationships with community.

These examples from Kenya and Australia represent the more
extreme end of the spectrum of healthcare contexts around
the world in which value-based healthcare is being adapted and
applied. However, all systems must weave value-based healthcare
approaches into their existing cultural and structural healthcare
contexts if they are to succeed. It never goes well when we seek
to impose our beautifully designed solutions onto somebody
else's world. During the course of the work undertaken in Wales
I have continually been struck by the similarities with the adaptation processes in other healthcare systems. For example, in
Saudi Arabia the Saudi Value in Health Centre (led by Dr Reem Al
Bunyan) has a strategic approach that is almost identical to that
in Wales. In the public healthcare system there, the Saudi Value
in Health Centre works closely with colleagues at the Centre for
National Health Insurance; and in the private system, it has a similar arrangement with the Council of Health Insurance.

While the drivers for value-based healthcare in public and
private systems are clearly different, the focus on measuring
and using patient outcomes in care and design of services is
ubiquitous. Saudi Arabia has universal health coverage, and I
was struck by the ambition to weave value-based healthcare
principles into the design and delivery of the so-called model
of care, meant to integrate primary care and population health
into local health clusters. Again, this approach encompasses a
diversity of needs and landscapes, from remote desert settle-
ments to packed urban areas, and the potential for high-tech
solutions in de novo healthcare systems such as that at Neom.[7]

Avoiding assumptions about care delivery: radical transformation

It is easy for us to assume that the way in which healthcare is currently being delivered is the only way and the best way. One of my favourite examples of why we should always challenge ourselves on the status quo comes from Cardiff and Vale University Health Board and their implementation of a novel approach to osteoporosis care.

Osteoporosis is a common condition, especially among older women, and it can lead to spinal and hip fractures. These fractures have a significant impact on a person's quality of life, and in the case of hip fractures, there is even a risk of dying. When I was a GP, I used to dread explaining the drug regime for preventing fractures to people with osteoporosis because the oral medicines were really unpleasant to take. I am sure most people failed to take them reliably because of that – and frankly, I don't blame them. I'm not sure I would have done so either.

However, in recent years treatment has been revolutionized by a monthly injection of a drug called denosumab. As this drug was introduced, the healthcare system in Wales defaulted to nurse administration of the drug, either in rheumatology outpatient departments or in primary care. Either way, this was a significant use of nursing time (and one must remember that multiple innovations in care are happening simultaneously, further crowding the clinical schedule). The health board in Cardiff consulted with patients and found that many were keen to be taught self-administration of the injection, significantly improving treatment adherence and patient experience and releasing huge amounts of clinic time to be spent with other patients who needed face-to-face care. Creative value-based healthcare in action, just as we saw in Kenya.

Palliative care: a special case

The clinicians who come to speak with me most frequently at the end of a conference keynote or presentation are palliative care physicians. This is true everywhere in the world. Typically, they open with something like, 'You talked about palliative care in relation to value-based care and the whole patient pathway! Thanks!' Along with geriatricians, primary care physicians and allied healthcare professionals, I have found palliative care specialists to be the most focused when it comes to eliciting and then achieving the outcomes that matter to people. This is of paramount importance as people approach the end of their lives. Maximizing quality of life and ensuring a peaceful death in a location of our choosing are as important outcomes as any others. As we saw in the previous chapter, it can be challenging to identify the right moment at which to discuss palliative care, especially for somebody with a non-cancer diagnosis such as advanced heart failure, liver disease or renal disease.

One of the projects that the Welsh Value in Health Centre supported was the work of Dr Clea Atkinson, a palliative care consultant who set up joint clinics with a cardiologist to provide shared care to patients with heart failure making this transition.[8] It meant that sensitive conversations about treatment goals and the wishes of patients and their families could take place in a timely fashion, improving access to palliative care and reducing the types of crises already identified as major problems by our ambulance service. So successful was this approach that it was soon expanded to people with end-stage renal and liver disease. These are the types of service innovation that get very little airtime at a system level but that are critical for meeting the changing needs of our populations, for improving outcomes and for promoting healthcare system sustainability.

Unicorns: value-based healthcare applied to primary care and urgent care

A common question I encounter is how to implement value-based healthcare in primary care. My view is that this is the wrong question to be asking, although it is certainly true that high-quality primary care plays a pivotal role both in improving the outcomes that matter *and* in reducing system costs. But primary care is a service. Value-based healthcare thinking encourages us to address the needs of patients with either the same medical condition or similar characteristics across an entire pathway of care. This means that no service can achieve value on its own: it can only do so by playing its part optimally in that pathway, in collaboration with other services.

Primary care provides 'first-contact' services to those with urgent care needs, chronic disease management, holistic care of older people, and a contribution to community palliative care. Primary care also plays a key role in diagnosing disease. Gaining an understanding of primary care's role in value-based healthcare requires us to understand the activities we wish primary care to undertake, how we measure the related outcomes, and how we reimburse primary care to support these activities.

A better question about value-based healthcare in primary care might therefore be: what role can primary care play in a high-value heart failure, diabetes or musculoskeletal disease pathway? And how do we measure that alongside patient outcomes? Following this line of thinking enables us to see that primary care is a key stakeholder in the integration of patient care and in bringing it closer to patients' homes: the so-called left shift that so many healthcare systems are trying to achieve. In other words, high-value primary care starts with segmenting patient need then integrating with other care providers across the pathway to provide a seamless experience for patients. If we can achieve this, we will truly understand value across the entire continuum of care.

Similar questions arise when we consider urgent and emergency care. Like primary care, emergency services provide 'first-contact' care for a diverse and heterogeneous group. Segmentation of the presenting caseload into people with similar needs is necessary here too, as we will see in the ambulance/palliative care case in chapter 7 when we discuss the importance of data triangulation in helping to solve wicked healthcare problems. An important case study in relation to urgent and emergency care relates to improving outcomes for older people. It is in response to this need that ICHOM set up a working group to develop a standard set of outcome measures that matter to older people. These measures include outcomes such as clinical status, disutility of care (polypharmacy and falls), quality of death (preferred place of care), autonomy, loneliness, pain, mood and impact on carers.

One of the challenges facing healthcare systems today is how to care for changing demography and the growing number of older people in our communities that are living with frailty. What do we mean by frailty? The British Geriatric Society say this:

> Frailty is a distinctive health state related to the ageing process in which multiple body systems gradually lose their built-in reserves... Older people with frailty are at risk of adverse outcomes such as dramatic changes in their physical and mental wellbeing after an apparently minor event which challenges their health, such as an infection or new medication.

When expressing preferences related to their care, many older people living with frailty express a wish not to be admitted to hospital. And yet, when a crisis – such as a fall, an infection or an exacerbation of a chronic disease – occurs, these patients are frequently conveyed to hospital by ambulance and then admitted. Why is this so? It can be a way of trying to manage perceived clinical risk; a mistaken belief that hospital is always the safest place to be; or simply a shortage of staff, skills or facilities to meet a patient's needs in caring for them at home. This latter scenario was something I witnessed multiple times as a general practitioner and it is very distressing to observe. 'Hospital-at-Home' has become a popular concept to address this difficult conundrum, and I believe this can be further supported through the measurement of ICHOM's outcome set that relates to what matters to older people living with frailty.[9]

We must remain cognisant of the fact that people living with frailty decondition frighteningly quickly when they are put into a hospital bed, and many do not regain previous levels of functioning as a result. For them, hospital admission is not a benign intervention, no matter how well-intentioned. It is important that we understand what matters to people and that we provide systemic support to healthcare professionals managing the risks of carrying out their wishes.

There are two essential parts to achieving this through value-based approaches. First, outcomes measurement, such as the ICHOM older adult standard set. And second, a detailed understanding and provision of the skills required for community teams to look after people under the Hospital-at-Home concept. Digital monitoring has a role to play as part of 'Hospital-at-Home', but ultimately the composition and mindset of the community team are fundamental to making it work.

Given the importance of frailty and the speed with which deconditioning in hospital can occur, one of the interventions I was keen to support in Wales was the development of a deconditioning tool. This is a clinically and patient-reported assessment deployed when an older person is admitted to hospital. It was the brainchild of my nursing colleague Rachel Taylor, with whom I had worked closely during the national Covid-19 vaccine campaign. It is designed to identify deconditioning and trigger early intervention with appropriate nursing care to mitigate against the effects of, for example, wasting muscles and deficiencies in nutrition. Once fully validated with the help of my old friends at CEDAR, it will be a big step forward in improving the outcomes of vulnerable frail people when they must be admitted to hospital.

If we think about the top reasons for ambulance conveyance to emergency departments – which in Wales are breathlessness, falls and palliative care needs – we can see that segmentation of the urgent care caseload can lead to root cause analysis of the issues, with solutions developed to improve outcomes before crisis occurs. This type of intelligence can lead to the creation of highest-value pathways that reduce the need for emergency care and reduce pressure on emergency services, just as we saw with the palliative care example. Tackling flow through the hospital – good operational management – is necessary. However, high-value urgent care delivery requires segmentation, pathway-level analysis and the reimbursement of properly designed community structures. This is something that must be considered at a policy level given that in most countries, individual organizations will not be able to solve this on their own.

Key lessons from chapter 5

Transforming pathways for value

- Whole-pathway thinking is crucial: prevention, early diagnosis, treatment, follow-up and end-of-life care.

- High-value interventions often lie upstream (e.g. prevention), but they are neglected in favour of 'rescue' efforts.

- Services must be redesigned around the *needs of patients*, not just existing structures. This requires a blank sheet of paper and blue sky thinking. In general, people find this very challenging to do.

Supporting self-management

- Chronic care needs patient involvement; outcomes improve when support is aligned with patient needs.

- Tools such as P3CEQ and Diabetes Distress Q help identify gaps in support and care planning.

- Outcome data reveals hidden barriers and service gaps, enabling redesign of care around real needs.

Reducing low-value care; adopting high-value care

- Low-value care wastes resources and can harm patients (e.g. when it results in unnecessary tests or ineffective treatments). National efforts (e.g. the 'interventions not normally undertaken' list in Wales) help track and reduce such care.

- Adoption of high-value care must be prioritized alongside reducing waste (e.g. introducing new technologies in diabetes care).

Adapting value-based healthcare globally

Value-based healthcare principles are universal and can be applied even in diverse and resource-limited settings.

- *Kenya*: MomCare used mobile technology and community support for maternal mental health.

- *Australia*: Healthy Outback Communities focused on integrated outcomes-driven care in remote regions.

- *Saudi Arabia*: national strategy mirrors Welsh principles, adapting to local context.

Misconception about value-based healthcare in primary care

The commonly posed question of how to implement value-based healthcare in primary care is a flawed one. Primary care is a service, not a standalone solution; value is created across the entire care pathway, not in isolation.

Value-based healthcare should instead ask: what is primary care's role in disease-specific pathways (e.g. those for heart failure, diabetes and musculoskeletal disorders)?

Segmenting patient needs and integrating services across the care continuum allows for higher-value delivery and supports the 'left shift' (bringing care closer to patients' homes).

Urgent and emergency care challenges

Like primary care, emergency care must segment heterogeneous patient groups for better analysis and response.

Segmenting helps both to uncover root causes of emergency healthcare use and to design proactive pathways to prevent crises.

Systems-level solutions are needed

High-value urgent care demands

- caseload segmentation,
- pathway-level analysis and
- policy-level support for community infrastructure.

Isolated organizations cannot achieve this alone; it requires coordinated policy and system design.

Conclusion

Implementing value-based healthcare in primary and urgent care requires

- focusing on patient needs and outcomes across pathways;

- promoting integration and segmentation;

- investing in community capacity, skills and reimbursement structures; and

- designing systems that deliver personalized, proactive care, especially for the elderly and frail.

CHAPTER 6

True north: driving value for populations

'Leadership is action, not position.'
— Donald H. McGannon

Understanding value in populations: choosing the many or the few

Value-based healthcare is a broad discipline. As we think more deeply about achieving value in health it is easy to become overwhelmed by the complex facets of healthcare and the multiple ways in which value can be achieved or lost. We often observe differences in the emphasis placed on addressing the needs and wants of individuals compared with addressing population needs equitably. All societies are somewhere on a spectrum between being a highly individualistic culture, such as that seen in the United States, and one that is highly focused on equitable outcomes for the whole population. The latter is often seen in government-funded healthcare systems such as the United Kingdom's National Health Service.

With finite resources, choices will always have to be made about how we manage this tension between individual needs/wants and population needs/wants, and every choice comes with a consequence in terms of an outcome for somebody – both negative ones and positive ones. I believe that a value-based approach helps us to take a balanced stance in addressing this Gordian knot because understanding the outcome data in sub-populations with the same disease or with similar sets of needs helps us to make better decisions about how to allocate resources effectively and fairly. By understanding variation in cost and outcome data taken together, we can also come to a better understanding of where we are investing too much or too little.

From an international perspective, approaches to universal healthcare such as that seen in the United Kingdom are sometimes criticized for leading to rationing. As societies we need to be clear. Rationing in healthcare exists everywhere in the world. It might be explicit, through government decisions on high-cost medicine adoption based on cost effectiveness, e.g. the recommendations made by the National Institute for Health and Care Excellence in the United Kingdom. Or it might be implicit, through high levels of out-of-pocket expenses for patients or through reduced equity of access to care. Nobody is exempt from the healthcare crisis. We need both value-based healthcare principles and political honesty with the public to help us chart the right course.

Macro-level decision making by governments has a significant impact on our ability to achieve equitable outcomes for our populations. This chapter is about nationally driven levers to achieve value in healthcare. It will explore approaches to decision making in the adoption of new technologies and other innovations. And it will consider the use of population data and financial levers in driving better outcomes and sustainable healthcare systems.

Value-based healthcare and decision making around innovation in medical devices

Any innovative intervention in healthcare should demand that we ask of ourselves what problem we are trying to solve, what the desired outcome is *for this individual*, and what the associated costs and ramifications are for the wider healthcare system. Nowhere is this more true than in the development and adoption of diagnostic, monitoring and therapeutic medical devices.

Health technology assessment is an important process. It is defined by the World Health Organization as, 'a systematic and multidisciplinary evaluation of the properties of health technologies and interventions covering both their direct and indirect consequences'. What we are seeking to do is achieve value both for patients, in terms of the outcomes that matter to them, and for healthcare providers and governments, who are under pressure to balance resource allocation to meet multiple needs of patients across the population they serve. Health technology assessment supports an evidence-based approach to that decision-making process.

However, an evidence-based path to the adoption of novel medical devices that might be of very high value to patients has historically been problematic.[1] We want to adopt novel devices and other innovations quickly and safely when they show a lot of promise, but we also want to ensure that they subsequently deliver on that promise in the lives of real people. We can and should back up our decision making with ongoing outcome data capture, including patient-reported outcomes, as part of real-world evidence generation. The push towards value-based healthcare is helpful in this regard as it encourages the embedding of patient-reported and clinical outcome data capture into direct care, thereby making it a more sustainable endeavour with the ability to create more robust datasets.

Many in healthcare are calling for a new relationship between industry and healthcare systems, particularly in considering new contracting models based on patient outcomes (value-based procurement). This should not be misunderstood: this new relationship with industry is not about driving the medical–industrial complex in isolation, without taking account of the impact of an intervention on the whole system of care for patients. We accept that industry must be profitable, but it has to provide value.

To achieve maximum value for patients we need to also ensure that we undertake two additional activities.

The first of these is, of course, to minimize unnecessary costs by adopting the most cost-effective product on the market. Careful attention to outcomes is necessary in order to make this judgment.

The second is to ensure optimal positioning of devices in the patient pathway. Does evidence-based medicine not achieve this? Examining data on device utilization from the 2019 NHS Wales Cardiovascular Atlas of Variation, it would appear not.[2] For example, the use of implantable devices for patients with advanced heart failure often correlates only with the proximity of the patient's home to the tertiary centre! Unwarranted variation – both overtreatment and undertreatment – exists, and we must tackle it. This is why data transparency is so important on a rolling basis. Unless we have access to the data, we are not alert to the problem.

Condition-specific patient-reported outcome data is essentially structured communication about symptom burden between an individual and their clinician. Having that data therefore provides information both about patient need and about the impact of an intervention on quality of life in a very specific way. Unlike generic measures of quality of life such as the EQ5D, it is generally harder to generate quality-adjusted life years (QALYs), which is the comparable measure of cost effectiveness that is usually employed by health economists as part of the basis for a health technology assessment. However, I would argue that these measures give us much more information about the specific impact of an intervention.

If we can both embed patient-reported outcome measures as a useful activity in the direct care of patients and find ways of using this data, including in the generation of QALYs from condition-specific tools, then we will enhance our ability to assess the value of medical devices and other innovations and to find their true impact on the lives of patients.

Another issue for decision makers in modern healthcare delivery – and a hugely important one – is the dawn of a new era of high-cost medicines and how we might afford them.

Value-based healthcare and decision making around high-cost medicines

We are on the cusp of a generation of medicines with the potential to cure or significantly improve outcomes for many diseases in ways we could not have imagined even a decade ago. An example of this is a group of medicines called advanced therapeutic and medicinal products (ATMPs). ATMPs include cell and gene therapies, and they might be used to treat genetic disorders, cancers or other long-term debilitating conditions such as macular degeneration, which causes blindness. There are a growing number of these products, as well as other medicines that are being developed to treat rare diseases. These medicines are often described as 'orphan' or 'ultra-orphan' drugs because of the very small numbers of people who will potentially receive them, and they are often very expensive.

The growing pipeline of high-cost medicines poses difficult affordability challenges for payers, and there is a risk that they will displace other forms of care or will hike the costs of healthcare insurance beyond the reach of the average citizen. Randomized controlled trials – the gold standard of evidence generation, telling us about the efficacy of medicines and therefore whether we should adopt them – tell us only so much about the likely outcomes from such exciting interventions. Value-based healthcare encourages us to think about our duty to measure outcomes on an ongoing basis after adoption, so that we can be sure the adopted interventions are achieving their potential.

In the 2021 paper 'Randomized controlled trials versus real world evidence: neither magic nor myth', Guido Rasi and his team said the following:

> In the future, specialized tertiary care facilities should be expected and held accountable to implement a high level of patient documentation that enables generation of high-quality real-world data, and ultimately the development of a 'learning health care system' with the ability to provide increasingly robust assessments of drug effects over time.[3]

They are talking about outcomes measurement, and implementing value-based healthcare, as a complementary approach to evidence generation alongside randomized controlled trials. Recognizing this, the Welsh Value in Health Centre recommended the funding and appointment of a permanent outcomes measurement director to the Welsh ATMP programme.

The difficulty we encounter is that current health technology assessment processes do not adequately assess the impact of a new therapy on the healthcare system. In publicly funded and capitation-based systems such as that in the United Kingdom, this means that as we adopt high-cost interventions, something else is displaced to allow us to pay for it. That displacement is frequently invisible, and what is being lost might be high-value care. Certain other services will become unavailable. In insurance-based systems, the cost pressure will fall on the insurer, and we will start to see exclusions or significant co-pays by patients. In all cases there will be growing inequity. No healthcare system in the world is immune from the impact of rising costs. Furthermore, these amazing new treatments will pose logistical challenges and require significant investment in infrastructure, particularly in tertiary (highly specialized) hospitals given the intensive care needed for many patients receiving these therapies.

To cope with these proliferating advances in medicine, healthcare payers will require new funding mechanisms to support the adoption of ATMPs and other expensive technologies. These will entail a degree of risk sharing between payer and supplier, based on outcomes achieved.[4] Organizations and healthcare systems implementing value-based healthcare will already have the infrastructure needed to collect the necessary outcome data to support innovative contracting after the adoption of these high-cost medicines, which is crucial if we are to ensure value for money.

When we started implementing value-based healthcare in the Aneurin Bevan Health Board, Adele and I had no idea about the far-reaching nature of the work we were doing. I certainly did not expect it to become a national movement. From a personal perspective, there were so many gaps in my knowledge – I even had to look up the word 'procurement' when I was introduced to Adele as I was not too sure what she did! But we learned as we went along, and I had many great teachers from the world of health economics and health technology assessment, from the life sciences industries and from procurement, all of whom helped us pull together the necessary strands of value-based healthcare at that macro level. The first and most enduring of these teachers was Imran Farid, with whom Adele and I tried to get several industry partnerships going over the years with the aim of improving care.

Imran Farid: the industry perspective

Imran Farid has worked in the medical technology industry for 20 years, applying his studies in theoretical health economics to the 'real-world' environment of the life sciences industry. Imran and I met in the very early days of the work that Adele and I were doing at the Aneurin Bevan Health Board. I recall having a cup of coffee with him in the education centre of one of our district general hospitals while he described a project he was supporting within the organization. Imran described having been introduced to value-based healthcare way back in 2007. He had come to see it as a set of 'real-life' approaches to enacting more academic health economic theory.

'Enhanced recovery after surgery' describes a tightly coordinated set of care processes that help people recover more quickly from a surgical procedure. Generally, it aims to reduce post-operative pain, to return a person to eating and drinking (and peeing and pooing) as quickly as possible, and to reduce the rapid effects of deconditioning that we see when somebody is confined to bed. As a result, the approach creates better outcomes and reduces costs, especially through length of hospital stay. So powerful is it as a part of value-based healthcare that I have always been a little surprised it is not more strictly adhered to by hospital teams.

Imran is a deeply principled man for whom I have a lot of respect. His observation of the global medical technology industry and his knowledge of international healthcare systems have led him to conclude that we are all on an unsustainable path, where rising costs will lead to unaffordability and a stifling of innovation in new medicines and other technologies. I asked him what he thought should happen now to mitigate against the major challenges we are all facing, and straight off the bat he gave me the following compelling analysis.

First, if we are to avoid rising inequity of access, worsening outcomes and greater restrictions on access to certain therapies, it is essential that we foster collaboration between healthcare providers and industry, and between industry and government, to build infrastructure and find novel solutions across healthcare pathways. Remember that all systems are facing the same challenges regardless of whether they are funded through taxation or are insurance based, private or public. It will not be long before insurance schemes become unaffordable: claims will become greater and greater in volume and magnitude, and then premiums will get higher and higher until many cannot afford them. Meanwhile, healthcare systems such as the NHS have insufficient capital to build the necessary infrastructure to cope with even current demand.

Second, we have to incentivize better health and view health generation as an important issue in terms of GDP and the economy. Health and healthcare must become everybody's responsibility, and value in health should be of interest to us all.

Finally, Imran said, we should get rid of the notion that everybody is doing value-based healthcare! What did he mean by this? Here, I believe he is reflecting on the dangers of a misappropriation of value-based healthcare by those who may have given it a cursory look. Value-based healthcare is about both improving outcomes that matter to people and managing our resources – not one or the other of these but both.

What population-level surveys tell us about value-based healthcare

Information from patients and the public at a macro level is an invaluable resource for helping healthcare systems design sustainable systems with better outcomes. It is for this reason that, in the summer of 2019, a small delegation of us travelled from Wales to the OECD head offices in Paris having been invited to participate in the first iteration of the new PaRIS survey. This was highly unusual given that Wales does not have a seat at the table in its own right – it is usually represented by the United Kingdom's Westminster government. However, in recognition of our growing work in value-based healthcare, the OECD had kindly invited us to take part and present to the organization's health committee. I felt huge pride for Wales as a little handwritten 'PAYS-DE-GALLES' sign was hastily scribbled and we took our place alongside the other representatives around the gigantic horseshoe of tables.

PaRIS, the first population survey of its kind in the world, examines patient-reported outcomes and experiences of those 45 years old and above. Essentially, it is measuring how well we are meeting people's needs in the communities where they live. We know that more people are living longer but not necessarily better lives as they struggle to cope with an increased burden of chronic disease over many years. This is evidenced in the PaRIS report by the WHO-5 wellbeing scores.[*]

Why is this an important finding? Apart from the human impact, this means that we need to configure healthcare in a radically different way. The patients who gave up 30 minutes of their time to respond to the PaRIS survey have told us what they need to thrive and to manage their conditions well, including how they need to interact with healthcare.

Access to a trusted professional, sufficient time with that professional, and continuity of care are all linked to better outcomes in primary care, and better outcomes in primary care are linked to reduced costs and to increased sustainability of the whole healthcare system. Investing in time and continuity of care is not, therefore, a soft option. In Wales, the current transactional approach of 'signposting' people with complex problems around an increasingly bewildering landscape of options might not be the best approach for people with lower levels of confidence about managing their health. It is a well-intentioned attempt to manage rising demand for services, but it is ineffective. I would also suggest that dwindling investment in chronic disease management and in sufficient time to do that well has also contributed to our poorer outcomes. It is sobering to see that Wales has the lowest scores of the 19 countries surveyed for social functioning and wellbeing despite being closer to average when it comes to the self-reported scores for physical and mental health. Fundamentally, the things we are doing to

---

[*] WHO-5 is a five-question survey that enquires after mental wellbeing and people's ability to have an active and fulfilling life.

manage demand are not meeting need. And worse than that, what we are doing can actually cause what is known as 'failure demand' within the system and contribute to system pressure and unsustainability.

Failure demand is defined by John Seddon as 'the demand placed on the system, not as a result of delivering value to the patient but due to failings within the system'. Two examples would be sending a patient to the wrong place or not having time to meet all of their needs during a chronic disease appointment. There is an awful lot of it about. It is often invisible to decision makers, and it is low value in every sense of the word.

The OECD report that came out of the PaRIS survey consistently shows that there is a correlation between better outcomes and (a) having adequate time with a trusted healthcare professional, (b) care tailored to the individual and (c) 'trouble-free' care. Workforce is also an increasingly precious commodity, so their time must be used where it adds most value and the use of digital tools should be accelerated to support patients where they can use them.

What does PaRIS measure?

PaRIS measures patient-reported outcomes across five domains:

- physical health,
- mental health,
- social functioning,
- wellbeing and
- general health.

It also measures patient-reported experience across five domains:

- confidence in self-management,
- experience of care coordination,

- person-centred care,
- quality of care experienced and
- trust in the healthcare system and professionals.

For this survey and for the population segment examined, there was a significant correlation between experience of care and outcome. This is unsurprising, given that for patients with multiple chronic conditions, confidence in self-management and having the tools to support that, experience of person-centredness and care coordination are all very important. I was struck by this quote from the survey report: 'People with multiple chronic conditions are usually expected to coordinate their appointments, integrate recommendations from different healthcare professionals, manage medication use and navigate the healthcare system.'

Less than half the patients surveyed in Wales feel confident in managing their health despite very high scores in supplying written information and in making referrals to relevant groups to support self-management. There is clearly something else missing then. Is it that patients need more time for individual coaching and care planning? Are we producing information in the right format?

Wales also scores less well on patients' experience of care coordination. We need to understand this in the context of emerging models of primary care in the United Kingdom. What the system thinks patients need and what they actually need might be different. Have we made access too disjointed, impersonal and transactional? It is encouraging to hear of plans to incentivize primary care to focus on continuity of care for this vulnerable group. Done in the right way, and measured with the right outcome measures, this could be a very positive move to improve on the current statistics in this report. To be clear, this is systemic failing, not a failure of healthcare professionals. It is also worth noting that we have a diverse multidisciplinary team in Wales, as recommended by the OECD, so this is not the problem. We do, however, need far more digital tools for patients to support their chronic disease management – something I have been arguing for as a priority for digital development nationally for some time.

And what about value-based care? Why has the Welsh focus on value-based healthcare not reflected in the PaRIS survey outcomes?

The answer to this is quite straightforward. The focus of value-based healthcare in Wales has to date mainly been in the hospital setting, and where it has been implemented, we have seen improvements in outcomes and costs. The PaRIS survey report highlights that the greatest value for patients lies in the community. It lies in exemplary chronic disease management (including supporting patients), prevention and early access to diagnostics. It lies in supporting the role of primary care in pathways of care. We now need to shift focus in Wales to this part of the pathway, and to enable this we need to modernize data policy to facilitate operational data sharing across the whole pathway of care. Doing this transparently will enable us to see where resource allocation needs to be prioritized and where behaviours need to be incentivized to drive better outcomes for patients and the population as a whole.

In short, we need to double down on value-based healthcare with outcome data transparency across the system, targeted investment and incentivization. At a national level, we need to obtain a feel for overall pathway costs – this is often challenging, but it is essential if we are to understand healthcare resourcing properly and improve outcomes for the long term. This is something we often fail to do given that decision making about resource allocation is often driven by targets rather than need. And it is one of the main reasons why – in Wales as in other places – there have been serial failures to meaningfully increase investment in primary care despite the rhetoric we hear about the need for more preventive and person-centred care that is closer to home.

Money is the answer: utilizing pay-per-performance, bundled payments, and capitation and incentives

From my earliest days working with Alan Brace in the Aneurin Bevan Health Board, I realized that the power base in any organization rests with finance. For good or ill, this is true of every organization that I have had interactions with. If finance wants something to happen, it happens. If they do not, it will be incredibly difficult to make progress. This is, of course, why Alan's intervention with value-based healthcare and outcomes measurement was so groundbreaking and powerful. He just made it happen by moving obstacles out of our way.

Just as finance are a powerful and influential professional group, financial levers are an important driver for value-based healthcare change. Value-based healthcare approaches to finance are intended to nudge people and organizations into behaviours that support both an improvement in patient outcomes and a reduction in costs. Incentive theory was first described in the 1930s by American psychologist B. F. Skinner. In his book *The Behavior of Organisms* he proposed the idea that human behaviour was not driven by internal motivations but by external factors such as expectations of reward or punishment.[5] As we saw with the Quality and Outcomes Framework for UK general practice in the early 2000s, financial incentives are a powerful tool for persuading professionals to do additional work to meet prescribed targets. Equally important is the reputational reward of achieving excellence. Incentives work.

In their book *The Patient Priority*, Stefan Larsson and colleagues describe with beautiful simplicity three broad categories of value-based payment.[6]

The first is pay-for-performance bonuses. These are payments for achieving a target or outcome.

The second is bundled payments. These constitute comprehensive payments to cover all activities in an episode of care or a pathway, and they are therefore a useful way of managing costs within that episode. Some portion of the remuneration is often dedicated to rewarding a specific outcome.

The third category is capitation. This is an approach that allocates a fee to cover all the health needs of each person in a patient population. In this model the healthcare provider takes on the risk, meaning that there is a strong driver for managing costs. In fact, unless capitation is linked to achieving outcomes, it can cause risk-averse behaviour that may lead to limitations in access to care that people need.

In Wales, healthcare funding from the government payer is underpinned by capitation, based on an allocation formula to the health organizations that is intended to be weighted towards greater need, based on a range of demographic factors. Within the allocation, funding is broken down into 'programme budgets'. These are notional budgets that are linked to individual medical conditions or to groups of patients with similar needs, such as around mental health. This payment model, coupled with the ability to oversee whole pathways of care in our integrated healthcare system, has great potential to deliver value for both patients and the healthcare system. Philosophically, the finance community in Wales conceptualizes value-based approaches to funding healthcare using a three-pronged model of allocation–utilization–outcomes. The model refers to the capitation formula (including the programme budgets or segments), analysis of the way we use resources across pathways of care, and finally the outcomes that are achieved.

However, we have yet to realize the full potential of this model. This is in part because we have rarely analysed the costs of care delivered against that programme budget segment, nor have we set those costs against outcomes achieved. We also lack two other things that are of behavioural importance. There is insufficient visibility of cost variations between the health organizations at a pathway level and a lack of specific payments linked to outcomes. The addition of total data transparency and outcome-related incentives should be the next step taken if we are to truly drive value-based healthcare to the next level in Wales.

The financing of healthcare systems is tightly bound to culture, history, legacy and politics in every nation of the world. It is unrealistic to assume that individual countries can adopt the same funding model for value-based healthcare. However, no matter what context we are operating in, we can think about how to apply the three funding principles of pay-per-performance, bundled payments and capitation to move towards systemic behaviours that favour greater value in healthcare. Indeed, we must do that if we are to have a chance at creating sustainable healthcare systems for the future.

The highest-value goal of all for the health of the population is a reduction in the prevalence of disease. For preventable conditions, therefore, it is logical to boost all activities that contribute to the reduction of risk factors. Fee for service is a common reimbursement mechanism in international healthcare systems that rewards activity, regardless of outcome. It is frequently criticized in value-based healthcare as being responsible for driving up activity and therefore costs, because as we know from incentive theory, what gets paid for gets done. As a colleague once said to me, if all prevention activity is good and desirable from the point of view of improving value in the long term, maybe we should make it fee for service!

Finding true north: governments must make the boldest decisions

The issues raised in this chapter cannot be solved by healthcare professionals or by provider organizations. They require big changes in policy to shift national levers in favour of achieving true value for patients, professionals and the healthcare system.

Healthcare is a political hot potato, and blame for the ills and challenges we see in healthcare today is often laid at the door of politicians. I have some sympathy for them, though: in the main, they are not responsible for the crises in healthcare that we see throughout the world. That said, while they certainly cannot solve these challenges alone, they will need to move away from glib soundbites about simple fixes that do not exist. Healthcare systems require radical and sustained transformation. There is no room left for short-term thinking. Policy leaders in health must keep a true north and hold firm on the direction of transforming healthcare even as political cycles come and go. Bold, technocratic decisions must be taken to enable better value healthcare.

Big potatoes

In my spare time I like to go trekking in mountain wildernesses. I love the physical and mental challenge, the rugged beauty of the landscapes, and the meditative focus that walking brings. However, there is always a point in every long trek when you question why you are doing it – when blisters appear and knees ache; when you feel you cannot go on. It is at that point you must dig deep into your reserves. This is when small things – a joke from a companion, a piece of chocolate or a beautiful sunset – can give you the impetus to put one foot in front of the other as you get closer to home. These testing points happen at work too, and large-scale transformation is a very long, very hard slog. To sustain ourselves we must be satisfied with small gains and words of encouragement.

Early in the value-based healthcare work at the Aneurin Bevan Health Board we were visited by a team from King's Health Partners in London. Heading up the team was a somewhat legendary respiratory physician called Professor John Moxham. I admit that I was a little bit terrified at receiving him in our slightly shabby office. However, when Adele and I reached the end of the presentation of our work to date – a presentation that we felt was wholly inadequate – the professor sat back in his chair and exclaimed: 'This is big potatoes!' We all fell about laughing. I never forgot that endorsement and encouragement from such a respected member of my profession, who had taken the trouble to travel to Wales to come and see us. I deeply appreciated the comment, and it sustained me through the hard times.

Key lessons from chapter 6

Tension between individual and population-level healthcare needs

Resource allocation must balance individual desires with population-wide equity.

Value-based healthcare provides a framework to manage this tension through the use of outcome and cost data across sub-populations to guide fair, effective resource allocation. It promotes transparency, equity and sustainability in decision making. And it recognizes explicit and implicit rationing in all healthcare systems.

The role of health technology assessment

Health technology assessment is vital for evaluating new health technologies and interventions, and it provides evidence-based frameworks for assessing cost-effectiveness and outcomes.

Make sure to encourage real-world outcome data collection, particularly PROMs, after adoption of new technologies. PROMs provide specific, relevant data on the patient experience and quality of life.

Condition-specific PROMs are harder to quantify in QALYs, but they provide richer, more precise information and context for them.

Embedding these into care pathways makes outcomes tracking more sustainable and robust.

Responsible innovation adoption (devices and medicines)

Decisions on new devices or drugs must consider

- the problem being solved,
- cost and outcome implications and
- system-wide ramifications.

Innovations must prove value not only in trials but also in real-world usage.

Equity and variability in access and care delivery

Unwarranted variation in care (e.g. device access based on geography) signals misaligned resource use.

Transparency in outcome data is essential to detect and address inequities.

The challenges of high-cost medicines (e.g. ATMPs)

Advanced therapies offer unprecedented outcomes but carry extreme costs.

Affordability and sustainability are central concerns – especially, but not only, in public systems. Displacement of other valuable services or inequity of access to treatments are real risks and are often invisible.

The need for new contracting and funding models

Adoption of high-cost innovations requires

- outcome-based contracts,
- risk-sharing mechanisms and
- infrastructure for data collection and evaluation.

Value-based healthcare implementation supports these needs by building systems for ongoing assessment of impact and value. This will be essential in the future if we are to develop affordable, equitable and sustainable healthcare systems.

Macro-level levers for change

Governments and health systems play a critical role in driving innovation adoption through policy and funding mechanisms.

Financial levers drive change. True system change requires finance leaders to shift funding towards value-based approaches.

Embedding outcome-based principles into procurement and regulation is desirable.

The emotional and cultural dimensions of change

Transformational work is difficult. Cultural shifts are sustained by small wins, by recognition and by encouragement. Symbolic affirmation can carry teams through long transitions.

A final message

Value-based healthcare at scale means seeing the whole system, valuing patient outcomes over activity metrics, investing upstream, and using data transparently and equitably. It requires leadership, vision and the courage to act on what matters most.

PART III

LESSONS ON INFRASTRUCTURE

CHAPTER 7

Turning data into wisdom: the foundation of value-based decisions

'Data is not information, information is not knowledge, knowledge is not understanding, understanding is not wisdom.'

— Clifford Stoll

Data, transformed into actionable information, is a necessity for value-based healthcare. Without it, we are unable to make informed decisions about care delivery; we cannot know our patients' outcomes; and nor will we understand how we are using our precious resources. This chapter explores the data requirements for value-based healthcare, and how we set about satisfying that need.

Why do we need data for decision making in healthcare?

'Data' is defined in the Oxford English Dictionary as follows: 'A collection of facts or organized information, usually the results of observation, experience, or experiment, or a set of premises from which conclusions may be drawn. Data may consist of numbers, words, or images.' Importantly, data is usually a collection of raw facts, figures or images that needs to be organized, structured and contextualized to give us meaningful and reliable information. Used out of context, data can also lead us to draw erroneous conclusions. But without data, we cannot generate the insights we need to inform us about what to do.

One of the fundamental tenets of value-based healthcare is the need for data-driven decision making. Specifically, the information that we use to inform our decisions at all levels of healthcare should include actual patient outcomes that matter (clinical and patient-reported). Equally important is the triangulation of clinical data points with costing and process data. Actionable information is important to everybody, so focusing on data quality and security, information governance and data interoperability should be a prime concern for everyone working in healthcare. In short, access to high-quality data should be everybody's business in healthcare.

Unfortunately, it is common for this not to be the case. An organization's lack of enthusiasm and/or understanding of issues relating to digital and data infrastructure results in underinvestment and an inability to access information that will support performance. This is particularly true of patient outcomes and patient-facing technology, and this is an urgent problem that needs to be solved in the pursuit of value in healthcare.

When I attended the value-based healthcare course at Harvard in December 2015 and was taught the principles of value-based healthcare under Bob Kaplan and Michael Porter, I quickly realized that datasets on outcomes and costs relating to care were, unfortunately, usually – in fact, almost always – absent from decision making in healthcare. This was true of clinical decision making with patients, such as guiding a patient towards deciding whether to take a treatment based on the outcome it might help them achieve. And it was also true of organizational and national policy decisions about how to allocate resources, incentivize good practice or understand whether the healthcare system was meeting the needs of its population. The necessary data was absent from clinical pathway design and, worryingly, patient outcomes were not the top priority when it came to assessing health system performance. In my experience the priority was nearly always financial performance and process metrics – the latter frequently relating either to waiting times to access healthcare or to length of stay in hospital. While these time-based metrics are important markers of a healthy system, they provide no information about how to meet patient need or, therefore, how to tackle demand in the system. Root cause analysis using outcome data would enable the design of longer-term solutions. Let me illustrate with an example.

The power of outcome data

An increasing problem seen around the world is the sight of ambulances queuing up outside hospital emergency departments. This can cause delays to patient care and increase the likelihood of an adverse outcome. Part of this problem relates to how well hospitals manage 'flow' through their departments and the timely discharge of patients back home. However, the increasing pressure on emergency departments also represents systemic failure to meet the needs of the growing number of people living with severe, chronic ill health in the community.

Unless all the necessary data to understand the nature of the entire problem is drawn together, the increasingly frantic attempts to apply a sticking plaster to the issue by making the hospital system more productive (i.e. making it go faster and harder) will ultimately be futile as demand grows. As ambulances are left stranded outside hospitals, ambulance services may be less able to respond in a timely way to emergency calls. Harm happens.

We gained some insight into possible solutions to this challenging system problem when we created a data dashboard for the Palliative Care Network, looking at outcomes for people who had been conveyed to emergency departments by ambulance in their last year of life. By fostering a collaboration between the network and the Welsh Ambulance Service, we were able to demonstrate that people with palliative care needs were in one of the top three segments of the population being conveyed to emergency departments by emergency ambulance.

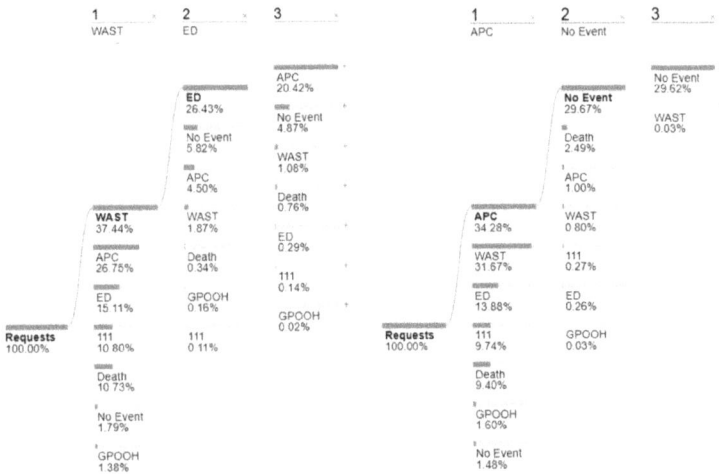

Left diagram — columns: **1 WAST**, **2 ED**, **3**

Requests 100.00%

1 WAST	2 ED	3
WAST 37.44%	ED 26.43%	APC 20.42%
APC 26.75%	No Event 5.82%	No Event 4.87%
ED 15.11%	APC 4.50%	WAST 1.08%
111 10.80%	WAST 1.87%	Death 0.76%
Death 10.73%	Death 0.34%	ED 0.29%
No Event 1.79%	GPOOH 0.16%	111 0.14%
GPOOH 1.38%	111 0.11%	GPOOH 0.02%

Right diagram — columns: **1 APC**, **2 No Event**, **3**

Requests 100.00%

1 APC	2 No Event	3
APC 34.28%	No Event 29.67%	No Event 29.62%
WAST 31.67%	Death 2.49%	WAST 0.03%
ED 13.88%	APC 1.00%	
111 9.74%	WAST 0.80%	
Death 9.40%	111 0.27%	
GPOOH 1.60%	ED 0.26%	
No Event 1.48%	GPOOH 0.03%	

Figure 5. Comparison of patients with palliative needs accessing emergency care. Those on the left have no access to specialist palliative care (SPC) services while those on the right do. (Produced by Digital Health and Care Wales (DHCW) on behalf of the Welsh Value in Health Centre.)

The analysis of emergency care data that is shown in the above figure depicts the sequence of urgent care 'events' for individual patients with palliative care needs. Each subsequent event occurs a maximum of seven days after the last. There are significant differences between those patients who were able to access palliative care services and those who were not. For example, a 'WAST event' (a Welsh Ambulance Service Trust emergency ambulance) followed by an emergency department attendance and then an admitted patient care (APC) episode represented 21.1% of event sequences in patients that never received SPC. By comparison, the same sequence only represented 13.9% of unscheduled care event sequences in patients that received SPC in their last year of life. This data suggests that patients with specialist palliative care input are less likely to require emergency healthcare in hospital than those without, suggesting that their needs were being met at home and they were being cared for in their preferred place of care. This is a very important outcome that matters to most people at the end of their lives.

Furthermore, we were able to ascertain that those who were not accessing specialist palliative care were more likely to have a life-limiting illness that was not cancer and that they were often conveyed several times during their last year of life. This information was triangulated with outcome data from the Palliative Care Network around preferred place of care and death, which brought about a realization that it was more difficult for patients with these diagnoses to access community and specialist palliative care. Plans had been put forward to rectify this through earlier identification of eligible patients and an extension of services, but the triangulation of this patient outcome data with the ambulance data provided a powerful stimulus for action. For me, this was both value-based healthcare in action at a very human level at the most vulnerable time in a person's life and a partial solution to one of the most high-profile problems in urgent care today.

In my dual roles as a general practitioner and as the assistant medical director in the Aneurin Bevan University Health Board, I was familiar with the use of data to illustrate variation in care. For example, I had access to detailed analyses of the amount of every drug prescribed across Wales and how that varied across primary care practices. This was possible due to centralized access to prescribing data coupled with excellent analysis and data presentation from the pharmacy team in the health board. Disappointingly, the same scrutiny was not possible for prescribing in the hospital at that time.

I also had access to data on the volume of patients attending emergency departments in the board's hospitals. I had data on the number and type of patient referrals from primary care into hospital specialists, and I had time-based metrics such as length of stay in hospital and waiting times for outpatients, diagnostics and surgical procedures.

Much of the focus in my organization was on reducing unwarranted variation in care, i.e. variation that cannot be explained by either evidence or patient preference. But the truth is that we often did not know if observed variations in care were unwarranted because we did not have information on the outcomes our interventions were achieving. Neither were we considering the wider impact of an intervention, such as a prescription, on the subsequent cost of care across a whole clinical pathway.

Think about Janice, the patient we met in the prologue. If I, as her primary care doctor, do not have access to effective early interventions in the community, her symptoms are likely to worsen and escalate. This is a tragedy for Janice and will result in her care escalating and becoming both more expensive and less effective at enabling rehabilitation. I realized that without outcome data, we were talking about variation in care without fully understanding it. This flawed thinking consistently led to failures to sufficiently invest in preventive care or to meet the needs of care in the community. In a taxation-funded, single-payer system such as the Welsh National Health Service, a lot of the work to reduce unwarranted variation was directed at managing demand on services, e.g. reducing referral rates from general practice to hospital specialists, or at reducing costs, e.g. lowering prescribing costs by monitoring variation against organizational guidelines.

In other healthcare systems, this frenetic attention to managing demand on resources does not exist in quite the same way. Indeed, in countries where hospitals and doctors are paid for the activities of patient care in the so-called fee for service model, increased activity becomes desirable because it is profitable, regardless of whether it is necessary, successful or even harmful for the patient.

These are just two examples of how organizational and national context, culture and values affect the way in which the principles of value-based healthcare might be applied. What is universally true is that we must understand patient outcomes and costs if we are going to do the right things for our patients and if we are to create sustainable healthcare systems for the future.

Despite the lack of outcome data, it would be wrong to say that all the activity directed at reducing unwarranted variation in care was about reducing costs. At times it was also about improving patient safety and reducing harm. For example, in 2013 I led a project to reduce unwarranted variation in the prescribing of broad-spectrum antibiotics in primary care settings. Broad-spectrum antibiotics are antibacterial drugs that are active against multiple types of bacteria. The advantage of these is that when the source of an infection is not yet known, you are more likely to be successful first time in treating it. It is obvious why these drugs might be an attractive proposition.

Unfortunately, the approach comes with a significant and occasionally lethal downside. These broad-spectrum drugs are also active against normal gut bacteria, and the loss of large amounts of these healthy bacteria can allow the pathogenic overgrowth of a bacterium called *Clostridium difficile*.[1] This bacterium produces a toxin that causes diarrhoea and inflammation in the bowel. This is highly infectious and can spread rapidly in hospital settings, and in some circumstances it can be fatal to vulnerable patients. Rates of *Clostridium difficile* infection are tracked as a key performance and safety data point for hospitals in the United Kingdom.

The public health department had mapped rates of community-acquired *Clostridium difficile* infection alongside broad-spectrum antibiotic prescribing data in primary care, producing a heat map showing variation by practice. The premise of the project was to reduce unwarranted variation in broad-spectrum antibiotic prescribing by flagging every new case of *Clostridium difficile* to the primary care team and for them to audit the underlying risk factors.

Linking the primary care prescribing of these antibiotics and other risk factors to each incidence of community-acquired infection led to rapid behavioural change in prescribing. Previously, practitioners had not had patient outcome data (in this case the clinical outcome of a serious infection) linked to their prescribing patterns. Seeing your outcome data in this way brings things up close and personal, and it shifts risk assessment considerably. As a result, we saw rapid and significant reduction in unwarranted variation in broad-spectrum antibiotic prescribing. This is a critical factor in reducing the rate of *Clostridium difficile* infection in hospital and its associated harm.

Unfortunately, the data-driven approach was not continued in the hospital setting because, at that time, the hospitals did not have an electronic health record or even electronic prescribing, meaning that it was virtually impossible to collect all the necessary data. This meant that we were unable to demonstrate sustained reductions in *Clostridium difficile* infection, because a whole-system approach is needed to achieve this.

This story illustrates two important points that became salutary lessons for me later, as I started to think about the implementation of value-based healthcare. Firstly, data transparency changes behaviour and is therefore essential to high-quality and high-value care. And secondly, it is often insufficient for one group of clinicians, on their own, to create sustained improvement of issues that arise in the healthcare system. Data must be turned into actionable insights that influence wider organizational decision making too.

On my return from Harvard in 2015, I realized that we had to incorporate patient outcome data not only into clinical decision making but also at departmental and board level too – and ultimately nationally. The dawning realization that the implications of the absence of patient outcome data had not occurred to me in 20 years as a practising doctor was like a punch in the guts. I also reflected that we were drowning in data but starved of actionable information that would make it possible to make wise decisions that would improve patient care.

Another important experience I had of using data to drive improvements in care was through the Quality and Outcomes Framework (QOF) for general practice in the United Kingdom, which was instigated in the GP contract in 2003/4 when I was a new partner in a GP practice in Bournemouth in the south of England. As we saw in chapter 4, this framework was intended to reward general practitioners for improving the quality of chronic disease management. Primary care practices, in addition to funding through capitation, had a portion of income remunerated through the QOF. In the beginning, this meant

- creating coded summaries of the patient record;

- creating and maintaining disease registers;

- creating recall mechanisms to remind patients on the disease registers that their checks were due; and

- maintaining certain clinical parameters, e.g. managing blood pressure or diabetes to certain clinical targets.

The QOF was not value-based healthcare, and it had some downsides, as we saw earlier, but it did illustrate two related points very well: data transparency changes human behaviour and people work hard at things for which they are incentivized. The speed with which chronic disease management processes were improved because of the QOF was breathtaking.

Did the QOF improve overall outcomes? It is quite hard to tell, but it is interesting that as incentives have been eroded in recent years we have seen a drop-off in performance against key indicators in diabetes, for example. The problem, though, is that we were not really measuring patient outcomes fully, and certainly not as a driver for integrated care across the pathway through this mechanism. And when primary care identified a need, e.g. the need for greater resources to support self-management of people living with diabetes, they were not supported by other parts of the system to deliver that.

If we are to truly increase value for patients and healthcare systems, we must take an integrated approach to care pathways and understand resourcing across the continuum of care, not just in the hospital setting or in the primary care setting. All of it should be looked at together.

Using data to drive value-based healthcare: costing and outcomes

Costing and value

High costs that do not tally with the best patient outcomes matter. They matter because rising costs have a negative impact on patients' access to care and to new technologies, and therefore on equity of opportunity to achieve the outcomes that matter to them. In Wales, as we tried to adopt value-based healthcare thinking, clinicians were encouraged to have an understanding of costs just as finance professionals and managers were encouraged to have an understanding of patient outcome data.

Ideally, costing of healthcare for value should be done for the whole patient pathway. This is important as it is not possible for value to be created in a single service – it must be assessed in terms of the outcomes delivered relative to the investment in all possible interventions for a particular population, whether this is a finite episode of care such as a cataract pathway or the costs attached to a population living with a chronic disease such as Parkinson's disease. In the latter case, we can take a 'year of care' approach to the costing, considering all the interventions that a patient has required during one year of care. This must include the cost of complications and of unplanned, acute care as this enables the organization to see that it needs to pay better attention to resource allocation through more effective service design that improves outcomes.

In Wales we use two main methods of costing, and both are required to gain a full picture of the cost of care in relation to the outcomes of care.

The first is patient-level costing, which is defined by the United Kingdom's Healthcare Financial Management Association (HFMA) as 'allocating costs, where possible, to an individual patient'. Assigning costs to individual patients in a hospital provides opportunities for a much greater understanding of how costs are built up. The system that gathers this information is known as the Patient-Level Information and Costing System (PLICS).[2]

The second method is Time-Driven Activity-Based Costing (TDABC), which is defined by the HFMA as follows: 'A costing method used by some to improve the accuracy of cost estimates for processes and interventions. It requires organisations to estimate the staff, equipment and time for each step of a process, the total costs associated with the staff involved and the time a patient will spend at each step of the process.' This method is particularly useful when assessing human resources across a pathway and when looking at the impact on costs of variable numbers of steps in a pathway. In my experience these are things that organizations frequently overlook. TDABC is the costing methodology recommended in Porter and Teisberg's seminal *Redefining Health Care*.

When TDABC was carried out across all the cataract pathways in Wales, a 40% variation in cost was identified due to differing approaches to patient pathways. It is clear, then, that this data can be a helpful driver for change.

TDABC is a relatively labour-intensive method of costing and it therefore needs to be applied judiciously where it will have greatest impact. A blended approach of using both PLICS and TDABC is particularly helpful because, despite the fact that we often talk about clinical activity in terms of linear disease pathways, peoples' experience of healthcare is frequently non-linear and complex. Pragmatic approaches to costing are needed.

The costing community in Wales soon came to feel that applying TDABC to every scenario was overly onerous and simply did not represent good value. As with any data collection, it is important first to decide why you need the information and then to tailor the approach accordingly.

From an international perspective, the context of the healthcare system matters a great deal. In highly fragmented systems such as those found in Australia, the United States and France, it is very difficult to obtain costing information across a whole pathway of care, from prevention through to long-term follow up. Patients will have multiple healthcare providers and no single record of their healthcare. Integrating care, and understanding the total cost of care, is nearly impossible, so providers will therefore need to begin with a partial pathway view.

Outcomes and value

What is an outcome? Too often in healthcare what we describe as an outcome is not actually a true outcome – not from the perspective of a patient at least. Much of what we currently measure are merely indicators, proxies or process measures, often used as benchmarks of organizational performance. These are frequently time-based metrics such as length of stay in hospital or the time it takes to access care. These are important but insufficient, and our system of measurement must mature so that we are also assessing the success of healthcare against outcomes that matter to patients.

It is pretty amazing that healthcare systems have not previously measured outcomes comprehensively and systematically, and that they have certainly not incorporated patient-reported outcome measures into care. The closest we come to this is in the implementation of national clinical audits and registries. Where these exist, they tend to assess care for a given clinical condition against agreed standards and guidelines. Most contain some clinical indicators and, occasionally, some patient-reported outcomes (an example here is the National Joint Registry in the United Kingdom).

Audit and registry data is typically held and owned by an external professional body, not the healthcare provider, with the latter simply being provided with an annual report of performance against the relevant standards. The inability of health organizations to access the data in real time and link to outcomes and other data they are collecting results in an inability to make improvements in real time. The remoteness and the relative lack of transparency lead to inattention and mean that the achievement of good data quality is not universally supported. To make matters worse, there is international variability in the creation of audits and registries, and even where they do exist, there is a lack of standardization of the data. Correcting this would really raise the bar of expectation in terms of what healthcare should be achieving.

At the beginning of this section, I mentioned that the term 'outcome' in healthcare is rather ambiguous. It is often used interchangeably with 'outputs', or it refers to events that are not directly linked to the patient outcome, e.g. the number of people seen in a clinic in a day. It is therefore important that we define outcome in the context of value-based healthcare before digging into the detail.

An outcome is an event that matters to a patient. It could be an endpoint or a consequence of a disease and its treatment, or it might simply describe the symptom burden of a patient at a specific point in time. If we do not ask people what matters to them, help them decide on realistic health goals and then achieve those goals, we are surely failing in healthcare. As Atul Gawande says in his book *Being Mortal*:

If to be human is to be limited, then the role of caring professions and institutions – from surgeons to nursing homes – ought to be aiding people in their struggle with those limits. Sometimes we can offer a cure, sometimes only a salve, sometimes not even that. But whatever we can offer, our interventions, and the risks and sacrifices they entail, are justified only if they serve the aims of a person's life.

Given that the word outcome is used interchangeably to mean different things, it is important to define exactly what we mean in practice. To this end, Michael Porter has helpfully defined a hierarchy of outcomes that matter to people, and his three tiers are summarized below.[3]

Tier 1 outcomes refer to the degree of health or recovery attained, and includes outcomes such as whether a person has been cured of a disease and other clinical outcomes. Much of this data is collected already, albeit inconsistently, in audits and registries.

Tier 2 outcomes relate to the process of recovery and describe in much more detail the impact on an individual of their illness and treatment, including the time taken to recovery. These outcomes are of profound importance and are rarely captured. A good example of this can be seen in patients recovering from major surgery. Dr Claire Dunstan, one of my colleagues in anaesthetics, has described how her team were beginning to tackle this issue in pre-operative care:

When Margaret, a 68-year-old retired teacher, was scheduled for colorectal surgery, her biggest fear wasn't the operation itself – it was the recovery. 'I'm worried about the pain,' she told me, 'and whether I'll be able to get back to my normal life.' Her concerns were typical. Surgery is not just a physical event; it ripples through a patient's emotional wellbeing, mobility and daily activities. Yet, too often, the medical record focuses on surgical success rates and complication numbers, leaving little room for the patient's own account of their journey.

In anaesthesia, where the patient's perception of pain, nausea and recovery is central, PROMs are invaluable for assessing the impact on an individual and for gaining a better understanding of how to improve these aspects of care, thereby speeding up the process of recovery (and reducing costs, through reducing the length of stay in hospital).

This situation inspired Claire and the team at Cardiff and Vale University Health Board to test whether they could implement PROMs and build a system that could listen to patients such as Margaret at each stage of their surgical journey, turning those insights into better, more personalized care. They chose a collection of validated tools:

- EQ-5D-5L and EQ-5D VAS, to assess overall health-related quality of life; and

- the Bauer questionnaire, to capture anaesthesia-specific experiences such as pain, nausea and comfort.

These were integrated into a digital platform, enabling patients to complete them pre-operatively, five days after surgery, and again at three months.

Claire and the team were surprised by the extent to which patients experienced severe symptoms attributable to the anaesthetic after major surgery. For example, about half of the patients who were asked had experienced moderate to severe surgical site pain, while a fifth had experienced severe nausea. Drowsiness and thirst were also common side effects.

A striking finding was that severe post-operative pain was strongly linked to higher pre-operative anxiety or depression scores. Interestingly, pre-operative pain itself did not predict post-operative pain.

These insights are valuable in anaesthesia care. They provide a clear, structured way to capture the patient's voice, identify pain points – literally and figuratively – and inform targeted improvements.[4]

Tier 3 outcomes describe the degree to which health or recovery is sustained, including capturing the long-term consequences of therapy. This will become very important information to help people make informed choices about their treatments and care.

Complete outcome datasets are needed to measure the tiers, and they typically contain four domains:

- case mix variables,
- treatment variables,
- clinically reported outcomes and
- patient-reported outcomes.

All four domains must be brought together to achieve robust analysis of a big dataset that is properly risk adjusted. The approach and methodology adopted by the International Consortium for Health Outcomes Measurement is very useful here.

For many, value-based healthcare has become synonymous with the measurement and use of PROMs, so it is critical to point out from the outset that while PROMs have utility on their own in the consultation, for most other purposes they require linkage with other datasets, as discussed above, if robust analysis is to take place. The reason for the intense focus on PROMs is probably related to the fact that in terms of routine healthcare data collection, they are the new kid on the block. Many healthcare systems around the world collect case mix variables, treatment variables and clinical outcomes routinely, either through electronic health records or clinical registries. The tricky part has been to implement PROMs data collection in such a way as to make it meaningful for all use cases.

Implementing patient-reported outcomes in practice is much harder than just talking about it, and the truth is that nobody really understands just how hard it is until they have tried it. The value-based healthcare paradigm has created great expectations about the use of aggregated PROM datasets to benchmark and improve care, to inform outcome-based contracts and procurement, and to provide real-world evidence after the adoption of expensive new technologies. The following sections explain what we learned about the prerequisites for PROM implementation that meets all the different aims listed in the following sections, and they tell the tale of how we managed to persevere in the face of setbacks.

Understanding patient-reported outcomes

So what is a patient-reported outcome? We can think of it as a milestone or endpoint in a pathway of healthcare that is reported entirely from the perspective of the person receiving that care.

PROMs are measured using validated questionnaires that might focus on pain, quality of life, wellbeing or the ability to perform activities of daily living. PROMs are not new. They have been used extensively to assess the effectiveness and cost effectiveness of surgical procedures such as joint replacements and hernia repair. They can be generic, as with the EQ5D-5L quality of life tool, or they can be disease specific, as with the EORTC QLQ-C30 for lung cancer. Ideally, both a generic and a disease-specific tool should be used together as they have different purposes. Generic tools such as EQ5D-5L can be used to make comparisons between quality of life gains in different conditions, and they are used in health technology assessments by health economists with a view to informing cost-effectiveness thresholds in different countries. Condition-specific tools measure symptom burden in relation to a specific disease entity.

Writing in the *New England Journal of Medicine*, US physician Ethan Basch summarizes the findings of his paper 'Patient-reported outcomes – harnessing patients' voices to improve care' as follows:

> Recording patient-reported outcomes electronically in real time and allowing clinicians to review longitudinal [patient-reported outcome] reports can improve patients' quality of life, enhance patient–clinician communication, reduce emergency department utilization, and lengthen survival.[5]

We have not truly begun to utilize these tools to their full potential in supporting our patients, particularly those with chronic disease. In this context, the word 'outcome' might sometimes be something of a misnomer, in that we are not really looking at endpoints here but instead tracking current health status from the perspective of the patient. The specific purpose of doing this will vary from clinical scenario to clinical scenario, but essentially PROMs are a great tool to support meaningful shared decision making and to allow people to lead their own care. Condition-specific PROMs are a structured assessment of symptom severity related to a specific disease. Capturing this information can enhance communication and understanding between patient and clinician. This opens a range of possibilities for increasing value, not least in raising health literacy, supporting self-management and implementing asynchronous or remote-care models.

Recent research by Dr Basch and others confirms our anecdotal observations and conversations with patients here in Wales: using PROMs in a clinic setting can be a very powerful way for people to prioritize what they wish to discuss in the consultation and to broach topics that were previously difficult or taboo. Longitudinal tracking of PROMs and clinical outcomes can give a more accurate perspective on the impact of a therapy, e.g. on motor function in Parkinson's disease or on pain.

Later, analysis of aggregated real-world clinical and patient-reported outcome data can help patients and their clinicians better understand the trade-offs between the benefits and downsides of therapy in addressing their personal health goals. This data becomes an important adjunct to randomized control trial data tested on a population that might have had multiple exclusion criteria. It begins to answer the important question, 'What will happen to someone like me if I choose this therapeutic course of action over another?'

Moving beyond the consultation, PROMs data sits alongside clinical outcomes, treatment and case mix variables. Analysis of this dataset can provide insight into clinical variation. Clinical teams who regularly review their outcomes are more likely to share knowledge, improve and innovate. Where benchmarking is appropriate, comparisons can be made with other teams, organizations and countries.

The complete outcome dataset can therefore also inform where we need to invest in services to improve outcomes for patients and their experience of the healthcare we are providing. I emphasize 'complete' because it is important that patient-reported outcomes are not used in isolation for this function. Because value-based healthcare describes PROMs as a newer dataset for collection, and the implementation of PROMs in care is challenging, there can be an overestimation of their utility in isolation at an aggregate level. Up until now, we have not had the necessary informatics infrastructure to efficiently embed PROMs data capture in care, but this is a rapidly developing field and major progress has been seen since the Covid-19 pandemic in 2020.

As important as the technology, however, is how outcomes are incorporated into the direct care of people using healthcare. This is a cultural and behavioural shift in care for both paitents and their clinicians. All too often, PROMs data, where it is collected, goes into a black hole, and response rates to questionnaires that are sent out to be filled in remotely are low.

This information needs to be visible to and accessible by both patients and those looking after them if its true utility is to be realized. It needs to be seen as a tool that is as important for care as a blood test or a scan. If we do not use the information that we ask patients to send us, we cannot be surprised if they stop replying to us.

In addition to respecting patients by using the information they send us, the burden of measurement must be minimal. This will be challenging: there is the potential for people living with multiple chronic conditions to be bombarded with PROM assessments from every department. This means we will need smart technology to ensure that duplication is avoided – a real problem in countries where care is very fragmented across the care pathway.

Now let us explore the main ways in which PROMs data is used in the tracking of chronic disease and in episodic care.

The different ways in which PROMs data can be used

(a) Longitudinal tracking of chronic disease

(i) Prioritization of issues by the individual. One of the first things to be worked on when capturing patient-reported outcomes in this context is to develop the ability of patients to prioritize and rank the most important issues to be addressed in a particular consultation from their perspective. This is a useful aide memoire for the conversation, and it improves the patient experience, facilitating a two-way exchange of knowledge, expectations and goals. This also tends to facilitate the broaching of issues that are more sensitive and difficult to talk about – think back to the inflammatory bowel disease example we saw in chapter 4.

(ii) Supporting shared decision making. Tracking outcome data can also be useful when assessing the impact of an intervention such as a new medication. As data accumulates, we will have the ability to utilize 'real-world' outcome data in reflecting back to patients information that is better tailored to their own context (rather than the context of an idealized population studied in a randomized controlled trial). This contextualization aids decision making, enabling people to make choices that are more likely to help them reach their goals and to think about the trade-offs between two different courses of action.

(iii) Support new models of care. As described in the section on costing, we frequently identify cohorts within a population living with a condition. Each cohort has varying levels of need. As we will explore later in the informatics section, outcome measures (combined with the correct IT functionality) can form an important part of developing new approaches to more flexible models of care, e.g. virtual monitoring.

(iv) Triggers for key decision points. Longitudinal tracking of outcome data reveals trajectories of disease progression over time and can therefore act as a trigger or prompt for key clinical decisions such as when to discuss anticipatory care planning or intervene to prevent hospital admission.

(v) Needs assessment. At a service and programme level, aggregated outcome data allows for the identification of population needs. The characterization and quantification of those unmet needs aids both service planning, through the identification of the above-mentioned cohorts, and, crucially, the allocation of resources. Value for patients cannot usually be delivered by a single service and instead needs a system-wide approach, so the marrying up of costing and outcome data is important here. We can then tailor services to needs more appropriately, e.g. in separating out those with new diagnoses, those who are stable on maintenance therapy, and those with complex and high-level needs.

(vi) Larger datasets. Larger datasets can be further triangulated with costing and process data for benchmarking purposes to inform efficiency and effectiveness, and this is also important for monitoring patient safety. Longer-term collection of outcome data can also provide real-world evidence to provide ongoing assessments of the impact of new medical technologies – something that is critical if we are to manage the clinical and financial risk of adopting new devices and medicines in the future.

(b) Episodic care

For a finite episode of care, outcome data can also inform shared decision making, which is particularly important in preference-sensitive clinical scenarios, e.g. where an invasive intervention may be undertaken for symptom control. For example, as patients we should always ask our doctor what the likely outcome is 'for someone like me' when considering whether to start a medicine or have a surgical procedure.

PROMs data is already in use for looking at clinical variation and quality improvement. Aggregate data of this sort does come with a health warning, though: even when it is adequately risk-adjusted, it does not tell us everything about patient preferences or goals. In other words, in data terms, a relatively poor outcome score may reflect the result of informed choices from the perspective of the individual receiving care.

This paradox is beautifully illustrated in many scenarios in *The Book About Getting Older*, a wonderful book written by my geriatrician friend Dr Lucy Pollock. Through storytelling, the book explains how people feel about the trade-offs in decision making between length of life and quality of life, and it looks at the impact of the burdens of treatment versus the benefits. This is why ICHOM developed outcome measures that move away from just looking at a single medical condition and are more holistic in their approach to what matters. For example, the

standard set of outcomes for older people supports the coproduction of 'Goldilocks care': care that is just right for a person
– neither overtreating nor undertreating them.[6]

When we assess value across a surgical pathway, we make
an assumption that the procedure was 'the right thing to do',
i.e. that the same outcome could not have been achieved
through non-surgical management approaches that are both
less costly and less risky. High-quality care does not necessarily
always equate to high-value care. This is why we need outcome
data to help people make decisions.

Developing a framework for PROMs collection: working out the why, what and how

The use cases for PROMs described in the previous section are
now well known but in the early days of PROM implementation
in Wales this was not the case. Through our initial feasibility
project with ICHOM at the Aneurin Bevan Health Board, where
we had supported the clinical team to measure outcomes for
patients with Parkinson's disease, we had realized that implementing PROM capture was a much more complex behavioural
and technical challenge than we had at first supposed it to be.
This meant that in the Value in Health Centre we needed to create a facilitatory framework with which to engage clinical teams
around their outcome data requirements so that we did not
miss out important use cases, such as using a PROM to support
remote care or building a data dashboard.

The framework was very simple.

- **Why?** Why do you want to measure a PROM, and what other
  data do you have/need?

- **What?** Do you know what PROM tools you want to use and is
  there consensus across the country, led by the relevant clinical network? (We always suggested starting with the ICHOM

standard sets where they existed and moved the conversation on from there.)

- **How?** What technology will you need and what support do you have for local implementation?

- **So what?** What impact do you envisage from implementing outcome data collection? What are your plans for increasing value?

We quickly learned that if we did not tease out all the ways in which the team wanted to use the PROM, we ran into difficulties. There were often issues with linking the PROM to clinical outcome and other data for analysis, for example, and we experienced difficulty when trying to display the PROM in another system, such as the patient electronic health record. In other words, the 'why' informed the 'how'.

We had found that the best way to embed the PROM in the direct care of a patient was to use bespoke patient-facing technology, such as an app, coupled with a personalized text message from their clinician asking them to complete the PROM as an essential part of their care. Key to closing this loop was the ability of the clinician to see this information in the electronic patient record so that they could discuss it at the next clinic visit (or for added reassurance if the patient was remote). Unsurprisingly, if this chain of communication was broken at any point, it became impossible for the clinician–patient partnership to engage further.

The ideal scenario, then, is for the PROM data to be able to move across into the electronic patient record and for analytics within the app to show the patient trajectories of their PROM data over time. I remember thinking how obvious and elegant a solution this seemed to me at the time. I also remember assuming that it would be straightforward to extract the PROM data from the app and link it to other data for analysis of larger datasets, as detailed in the use cases above. I soon came to realize how dramatically I had underestimated the problem. I was about to be exposed to the world of data standards, interoperability and information governance. There is just no way to fully understand the implementation of value-based healthcare without getting into these tricky technical issues.

Overcoming digital obstacles: data standards, interoperability and governance

Digital systems in healthcare can be characterized as a plethora of individual digital services with different functions. In the Welsh NHS, as in its English counterpart, there are currently more than 100 of these services in operation. This is probably a conservative estimate. Many countries are not able to estimate how many individual digital systems are in operation across the healthcare system due to greater fragmentation within their system. Most of these systems do not 'talk' to each other, which is a constant frustration for patients, clinicians and data analysts alike. It is interoperability, enabled by the rigorous application of data standards, that allows digital systems to talk to each other. And it is information governance laws and guidance that grant or deny the necessary permissions for this to happen.

I mentioned in chapter 2 the importance of building boundary-spanning and multidisciplinary relationships to help solve wicked problems in healthcare, and here we can see two major hurdles to value-based healthcare: interoperability and governance. I needed help from my colleagues in informatics if we were to create PROMs data standards for Wales that would enable the implementation of value-based healthcare in a standardized way across the country and for later comparisons of outcome data to be made possible. I also needed help with national data sharing agreements for PROMs.

On a personal level, I found all this completely exhausting. At times it felt like an impossible mountain to climb. So much of my time seemed to be devoted to building and correcting infrastructure before we could even think about actually implementing value-based healthcare or the exciting healthcare transformation work that was so sorely needed by my patients and colleagues. Fortunately, help was at hand. Helen Thomas had recently been appointed to the role of director of information at the National Welsh Informatics Service, the precursor to Digital Health and Care Wales. She had been given the task of developing a strategic approach to developing a National Data Resource for Wales – essentially a single repository for all healthcare data in Wales. This was in response to a policy directive from the Welsh government: the 'Information Statement of Intent'.

Helen and I met at the Healthcare Information and Management Systems Society (HIMSS) conference in Malta in 2017. We hit it off straight away. Although we had followed very different paths in healthcare, we had shared values and a shared conviction that we could do so much better for patients if we adopted a more data-driven approach to decision making. I could see the potential of Helen's vision for a National Data Resource in supporting the aims of value-based healthcare by bringing together all the data we needed to better inform patient care: outcomes, costs, administrative data – the whole works. Helen could see that value-based healthcare provided an accessible rationale for the painstaking work that would be needed to develop the National Data Resource. This was the beginning of an important partnership.

Helen Thomas: forging a path through the data landscape

Helen started off her career in healthcare finance and worked her way up through the ranks. Right from the start she held a strong sense of purpose in her role, and she was soon attracted to data and to its importance as a tool for improvement in healthcare. This was work that mattered.

She quickly – and to my mind rather bravely – changed career direction to train in data science and business analysis. In her early roles in healthcare information she gained a deep understanding of how healthcare works. She understood the processes of care, behind the scenes, and she regularly worked with clinicians on the data that was coming back from clinical audit. Even in these early days, Helen was frustrated that clinical outcome data was usually submitted to external clinical audits and registries, analysed remotely, and then returned in a report to clinical teams and providers around 18 months later. How was this helpful for timely improvement in care?! The challenging but fascinating conversations about clinical data with clinicians were to become a powerful driver in her thinking about how data should be collected, stored, shared and turned into meaningful insights.

The flagship Prudent Healthcare movement, launched in 2014 by Professor Mark Drakeford (health minister for Wales at that time), was as significant a milestone for Helen as it was for me. She recalls being struck by how clear and brave a direction of travel this was, in wanting to improve outcomes and promote healthcare system sustainability. Also like me, Helen felt that while it was an amazing philosophy of care, it was insufficient unless we could attach measurement to it. In short, we needed data to support care, to support improvement, and to inform resource allocation.

As she settled into the national role as director of information at the National Welsh Informatics Service, Helen observed that we were 'data rich, but information poor'. Too much of our data was siloed or inaccessible, and there were too many arbitrary barriers to using it for the benefit of patients. She recalls thinking that value-based healthcare was the key to unlocking progress with the Prudent Healthcare principles, and to illustrate the importance of measuring and using outcome data for improvement. She now says: 'The use cases for value-based healthcare helped us explain information governance, helped people to understand why data sharing was important for patient care and how it could be done safely and appropriately.' It took technocratic and abstract concepts into the realm of the human and the relatable.

Helen was instrumental in helping me build the team inside the National Welsh Informatics Service/Digital Health and Care Wales. Our incredible little team have acquired raw data feeds back from the national clinical audits and registries and inputted them into the National Data Resource so that we can link this data to PROMs coming in from the health board teams. This will also link to our costing data. As this dataset grows it will provide amazing opportunities to analyse effectiveness of care and value and to generate real-world evidence to enhance our understanding of new medicines and technologies as they are adopted. In addition, it will support value-based procurement as we develop new models of sharing the risk of paying for high-cost therapies; this is vital if we are to prevent stagnation of innovation or growing inequities in access to technologies.

It was no surprise to me that Helen rose to be the chief executive of Digital Health and Care Wales when it was established in 2021. She reflects now that the value-based healthcare agenda is almost business as usual within her organization. Under her leadership, many more resources have been directed towards building the technical infrastructure for value. The improvements include progress on information governance and data sharing, the building of new data tools, and the taking forward of developments in patient-facing technology. Many members of the Digital Health and Care Wales workforce have rotated through the value-based healthcare team there. Helen is building a clinically focused team of analysts for the future.

A digital solution for Wales: a standard operating model for PROMs and a single gateway for patients

With value-based healthcare maturing, every health organization in the country came to have both a value-based healthcare team supporting implementation internally and patient-facing software to engage people in completing PROM assessments.

All of the teams were struggling with interoperability between their digital systems, and this was proving really frustrating for clinical teams who were not able to see their data wherever and whenever they needed to. The logical thing for us to do at the Value in Health Centre was to create a standard operating model for PROM collection in Wales: the PSOM.

The PSOM was devised by my chief digital officer Dr Said Shadi, an expert in data standards and artificial intelligence. In negotiation with the health board value-based healthcare teams, with software suppliers and with Digital Health and Care Wales, Said devised a specification for an ePROM system that met all clinical and organizational user requirements (see figure 6 on the next page). This alone was a considerable achievement, but Said went further. Working with the National Data Resource team at Digital Health and Care Wales, he and the value team set about defining PROM data standards for Wales and mapping to Fast Healthcare Interoperability Resources (FHIR).[7]

This painstaking work took two years to complete but eventually resulted in the procurement of an all-Wales PROM system that was data compliant and that would allow full interoperability with all the Welsh digital systems. It was also able to work alongside the growing clinical data repository in the National Data Resource, this having being built on OpenEHR standards.[8]

We had learned very early in our value-based healthcare journey that PROMs implementation should not be approached as a data-collection exercise. It is far more profound than that. It is about enhancing digital communication with patients, and it can be a fantastic tool for empowering people to take control

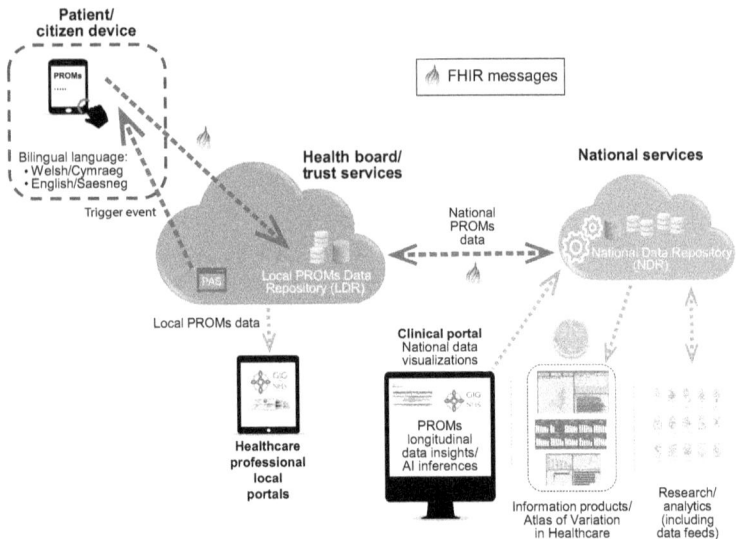

Figure 6. Creating PROM interoperability in the Welsh system. (Reworked, with permission, from an original diagram created by Dr Said Shadi.)

of their health information, for improving health literacy and for supporting person-centred care. Like many others around the world, we realized that this enhanced digital communication could support new and more flexible models of care. This was critical to thinking about sustainability, especially in how we made the most of precious clinical time at a time of growing workforce crisis.

When we began our work in 2016, this was a novel approach, but during the pandemic we saw an exponential rise in the development of patient-facing applications to support remote care and provide patients with information.[9] On the one hand this was a very positive thing, accelerating progress towards value-based healthcare and towards truly innovative and transformative approaches to healthcare for those ready and able to use these technologies. On the other hand, app proliferation could almost be described as feral: wild and disconnected from other digital systems. This posed risks and challenges in the areas of safety, cybersecurity and information governance, and it presented a confusing and burdensome interface for patients.

There was also the potential for economies of scale if we could rationalize the procurement of some applications at the national level. However, it was desirable for providers to retain control of applications that communicate with patients for reasons that I hope are obvious. People need to feel that they are in direct communication with their healthcare provider, not with an amorphous centralized data control centre. And we would never achieve person-centred care if services could not be locally configured.

To help organize my own thinking on this, I used the mantra 'communication is local; information is national'. In other words, we needed locally configurable software to support a close relationship with patients, but it always needed to conform with national data standards so that our digital systems remained interoperable and connected.

The approach described above is very easy to describe but very difficult to deliver. Digital Health and Care Wales decided to do something about it and created the Digital Services for Patients and Public Programme, which was meant to bring some coherence to the app landscape. Hamish and I joined the Board immediately, given our mutual interest in driving this forward in the right way. The biggest barriers to progress in achieving a degree of consensus in the Welsh digital community were twofold: deciding whether this was the right approach and choosing where to begin. It was critical to have that buy-in or the whole programme risked becoming a white elephant.

I was given the task of chairing a group of digital and clinical leaders to gain that buy-in so we could get started. This was the summer of 2020 and we were all reeling from the first wave of the Covid-19 pandemic. I decided to give us a deadline of three weeks to achieve – or fail to achieve – consensus. Six meetings later we had wobbled to a point of precarious agreement on both the approach and priorities – an important moment for patient-facing technology and for value-based healthcare in Wales. The roadmap towards digital services for patients became a critical component of the PROMs standard operating model: the ability for patients to access digital functions through a single gateway application. Essential protective functions such as cybersecurity and information governance were centrally owned by Digital Health and Care Wales, but other local apps could be 'plugged in' behind it, including the software to collect PROMs.

Developing a robust process for PROM oversight

As the number of requests from clinical networks for PROM implementation quickly rose, we also needed to develop some sort of quality assurance process to provide oversight to the selection, translation and analysis of PROMs.

Patient-reported outcome questionnaires (we like to call them assessments) compile carefully worded queries to patients about their symptoms and their quality of life. The questions are derived following a long research process during which they are tested and validated across patient groups to ensure that they are universally understood and interpreted correctly. It is essential to use validated tools and, in many cases, standardized timepoints for collection in relation to surgical procedures and therapies. Failure to do so brings with it the risk of deriving the wrong conclusions from subsequent analyses.

Wales is a bilingual country and there is a legal requirement to provide patient materials in Welsh as well as English. PROM translation was an essential part of our programme of work from the outset, and this is likely to be the case in almost every country in the world. Like validation, translation of a PROM into another language is a labour-intensive process. Essentially, the translation must be validated with focus groups of native speakers to ensure that the translation is a correct interpretation of the original question. Adjustments to account for different cultural contexts will also be needed.[10]

We realized that we needed expert help to coordinate the growing number of requests for PROM implementation from the national clinical networks so that we could maintain a robust process for PROM selection, the purchasing of PROM licences, PROM translation, statistical analysis and the validation of new tools where needed. We commissioned the services of CEDAR, a research institute that has excellent multidisciplinary skills and that could manage the entire PROM package. PROM implementation carries with it considerable costs and practical challenges, and again these issues will be universal in every country. How they are tackled will depend on the local context, on the degree of value-based healthcare adoption in the country and on the availability of in-house expertise (e.g. ICHOM support).

Everybody loves a dashboard, but data is not wisdom

With the help of my informatics colleagues, we began to chip away at the digital barriers to value-based healthcare implementation. Thanks to my deepening relationship with Digital Health and Care Wales I funded the creation of a team dedicated to value-based healthcare within that organization. One of the team's first tasks was to build national outcome data dashboards. My oh my, everybody wants a dashboard! The team began to build dashboards as a kind of standard reporting product or repository for outcome, process and (sometimes) costing data. They created them for a variety of conditions, from cancers to musculoskeletal and chronic diseases such as inflammatory bowel disease and heart failure; one of the most important was the 'last year of life' dashboard, which gave us a deep understanding of what was happening to people who needed palliative care.

Well, that's great, I thought. Now we have these dashboards containing rich datasets, clinically curated by subject matter experts in the national clinical networks. Now we can expect real change and an attention to patient outcomes across all healthcare providers in the country. But remember: 'Data is not information, information is not knowledge, knowledge is not understanding, understanding is not wisdom.'

Although we had arranged for everybody in NHS Wales to have role-appropriate access to all the data dashboards, hardly anybody in the organizations was using them on a regular basis to inform and track value improvements. We quickly realized that, on its own, data is not enough. To effect change, it needs to be transformed into actionable insights – and in my view, transparent and, ideally, public ones. It is also helpful if the data can be made visually appealing and digestible, so that large amounts of information can be quickly assimilated by people who are not data experts. If this is not achieved, not much happens at a national level.

The other problem we faced was a lack of incentivization and/or penalties to ecourage healthcare providers to focus on outcome improvement. In other words, there were not enough sticks and carrots to nudge behaviour. Sticky carrots, as I like to call them.

As I lamented the relatively disappointing impact of our national dashboard fetish, I remembered a lecture I had seen at a University of Oxford conference during my early days exploring value-based healthcare. Professor Sabina Nuti, a hugely impressive and charismatic lady from the Scuola Superiore Sant'Anna in Italy, was presenting her work on reducing unwarranted variation and the number of adverse outcomes in diabetes care. The Scuola, part of the University of Pisa in Tuscany, has a huge data lab. Over the last 20 years or so, the team there have run a voluntary programme with the Italian regions looking at healthcare system performance data.

There are two striking things about this data project. First, the data is published on their website and is public. And second, the team have extensively tested different data-visualization techniques with hospital managers to see which they prefer and which they can interpret most easily. They have come up with two particularly elegant solutions for presenting large amounts of data in such a way that it is very easy to see where there is variation in system performance and clinical outcomes. The solutions are based on a musical stave and a dartboard, and they enable anyone to derive meaning from extremely large amounts of data at a glance.[11,12]

I decided to get in touch with Sabina again to see if we could try to adopt some of the Italian techniques. The team at the Scuola generously invited our data team over to witness the work in progress first hand, and the trip resulted in a long-lasting collaborative relationship on data-visualization techniques, research and value-based healthcare education that endures to this day. We learned a great deal from our friends in Pisa but also quickly realized that we did not have the resources necessary to do the work at scale (the Pisa team was 60-strong). Neither was there yet an appetite in Wales to make this level of performance and outcome data public.

Key lessons from chapter 7

Data as the foundation for decision making in healthcare

Raw data ≠ useful information. Data must be organized, contextualized and interpreted.

Value-based healthcare requires actionable data. Data relating to outcomes, costs and processes must be triangulated and presented as actionable information if it is to inform decision making.

Poor digital infrastructure hampers the ability to utilize data effectively, especially for patient-facing technologies.

The critical role of outcomes in healthcare

Patient outcomes are often ignored in healthcare decision making. Financial and time-based metrics dominate decision making instead of what matters to patients.

Outcomes are needed at all levels. We should be using patient outcome data to inform decision making in the therapeutic consultation and in clinical pathway design, and we need to use it at a national level to understand healthcare system performance and population need.

True outcomes include patient-reported data, not just clinical indicators or process metrics.

Case studies in data use

Collaboration between different professional groups led to data triangulation and enhanced systemic understanding of patient needs. This approach supports effective problem-solving to improve outcomes and resource utilization.

Data transparency drives behaviour change; improving outcomes needs organization-wide engagement.

Using patient-reported outcome data

PROMs capture the patient's voice (symptom burden and quality of life) using validated tools.

PROMs have multiple uses in healthcare, as follows.

- They enable shared decision making in the therapeutic consultation.

- They make longitudinal tracking of chronic disease management possible.

- They are triggers for intervention.

- They highlight and codify patient need, both for individuals receiving care and, when aggregated, for sub-populations. The latter can inform service redesign to meet a given sub-population's needs.

- They also play a role in value-based procurement, e.g. of medicines and medical devices.

But PROMs also present challenges. People disengage with PROMs capture if data is not visible to clinicians and patients or if it is not used meaningfully. Therefore, embedding PROMs in direct care should be a priority.

Costing in value-based healthcare

There are two main costing methods:

- Patient-Level Information and Costing Systems (PLICs): these systems assign costs to individuals.

- Time-Driven Activity-Based Costing (TDABC): these track resource usage along care pathways.

A full-pathway view is needed. Ideally, it is necessary to build up an understanding of the costs of healthcare across the whole pathway of care if we are to avoid a distorted understanding of value.

Data implementation challenges

The PROMs Standard Operating Model (PSOM) in Wales was developed to standardize functionality and to ensure interoperability. Significant expertise is needed to overcome technical implementation barriers such as

- fragmented digital systems,
- data standards and interoperability issues, and
- information governance and data sharing.

Technology and integration

It is important that PROM data can be surfaced in the electronic health record. Being able to do this enables use during clinical consultations.

Dashboards can be useful for bringing together data and visualizing it, but regular use of complex information products is something that usually remains limited to enthusiasts. Actionable insights must be generated to support decision making.

A key lesson from the Pisa team in Italy is that visualization techniques and public data transparency can drive real change.

Data must lead to action

Data ≠ wisdom. Raw numbers must be transformed into understandable, digestible and motivating insights that can be acted upon.

Culture change is required. Without incentives or accountability, data is underutilized.

Overarching principles

- Transparency and engagement with clinicians and patients are key.

- Success requires system-wide integration of data, outcomes and incentives.

- Behavioural and technical barriers must be addressed concurrently.

CHAPTER 8

Passing the baton: what next for value-based healthcare?

'In the midst of chaos there is also opportunity.'
— Sun Tzu

Redesigning services is everybody's business

Too many presentations on value-based healthcare start from the assumption that the onus for higher-value care rests entirely on clinical teams to improve outcomes and costs. The belief is that those teams can achieve that goal through quality improvement in their service alone.

While doctors, nurses and allied health professionals are pivotal in achieving the best outcomes for patients, they have no control over other parts of the pathway, either within their organization or outside it. They have no control over whether new models of care are financially supported, whether that is by investment from a single government payer or by an insurance company's reimbursement model. Radical system redesign that meets population needs sustainably requires alignment between payer, provider and clinician. Achieving value in healthcare is everybody's responsibility, and it requires innovative ways to tackle fragmented service provision across the care pathway.

Value-based healthcare as a driver for integrated care

As I track the implementation of value-based healthcare across the world, I see many organizations that are doing their best to improve value for patients but are unable to 'see' the whole pathway because of a fragmented structure in their country's healthcare system. The result of this fragmentation is that care tends to continue to focus on the hospital setting, neglecting integration with primary care that is closer to people's homes. We need to take an international perspective and talk about the problem of fragmentation and how value-based healthcare will need to influence policy-making if this problem is to be corrected. A helicopter view of patients' needs is a necessity, and associated funding flows will need to be addressed if true systemic value is to be achieved.

The antidote to fragmented care is integrated care, which can be thought of as seamless and coordinated care such that the person receiving that care does not perceive any gaps in service or experience the need to keep telling their story over and over again. Integrated care means creating care around the patient, and it requires different stakeholders across the patient pathway to work together.

With its focus on whole pathways of care and a collective view on patient outcomes, value-based healthcare is a natural driver of integration in healthcare. Porter and Teisberg described integrated practice units (IPUs) as the solution to fragmentation of care in the US context. IPUs are generally co-located multidisciplinary teams that can organize care around the needs of a particular patient group, and they can be a very useful approach to care delivery for certain patient groups and for medical conditions such as rare inherited diseases or conditions that require a lot of specialist input. For example, we have IPUs in Wales for people with advanced renal disease and for people living with cystic fibrosis.

But IPUs are not the only way to successfully integrate care, and the way we think about integration of care is – as with so many facets of value-based healthcare – highly contextual. It is possible to integrate care across pathways of care with collaboration between different providers, and in some circumstances this is essential: where there are very high patient volumes and care closer to home is desirable, for example, or when we want to better integrate between the disciplines of primary and secondary care, and social care.

The important factors are that care appears to the patient to be seamless and, for the healthcare system, that the best use of available resources is made.

The pitfalls of implementation

One of the common pitfalls of value-based healthcare is to rush towards the implementation of outcomes measurement, and especially PROMs measurement, without first considering what change we might want to see. This can lead to PROMs measurement being seen as an end in itself. When approached in this way, PROM data is not actually used, which risks disengaging both patients and clinical teams. And as we have seen throughout this book, there are many operational activities that are necessary higher-value care that do not involve PROMs.

Work on organizational culture and strategy towards value-based healthcare must be carried out in parallel, with a focus on demonstrating impact right from the start. Otherwise, good people lose faith, and any early interest will soon peter out. The issue in this situation is not a failure of value-based healthcare, but a failure of implementation. No approach to healthcare transformation is a panacea, and value-based healthcare is no exception to this rule. However, as we have seen throughout this book, it is both a radical mindset and a toolbox for transformational change.

The second common error in value-based healthcare is to ignore the organizational and national context in which you are trying to implement it. Trying to impose an exact replica of a service model seen in another country, or attempting to enforce the same financial structures or incentives, is bound to fail. Successful adoption of value-based healthcare requires the application and adaptation of the principles in this book to the local healthcare context. We have to take people and the system on the journey with us.

Building a team – locally and nationally

Organizations implementing value-based healthcare need a critical mass of people who understand the concept and what it is trying to achieve. An organizational culture and strategy built on the foundations of value is key to success – it is an underpinning philosophy that is necessary for success.

A systematic approach to value-based healthcare education and engagement is therefore critical. There should also be a dedicated internal team to support the necessary change management on the ground, particularly in relation to the practical aspects of outcome implementation. This team should be multiprofessional and must have access to clinical, managerial, financial, digital and analytical expertise, as all these skills are required to achieve value in healthcare. We cannot solve the wicked problems of healthcare alone; we need each other.

My friend and colleague Dr Tara Sood, an emergency physician at the Royal Free Hospital in London, describes these multiprofessional partnerships as being 'where the magic happens'; I profoundly agree with her. Traditionally, there has been a rather adversarial relationship between doctors and managers, for example, which is wholly counterproductive to patient care. Value-based healthcare really can unite us in our focus on patient outcomes while simultaneously being good stewards of healthcare system resources.

The role of a national centre for value-based healthcare is to ensure that the correct infrastructure is in place for value-based approaches to succeed and to provide policy advice on the alignment of system levers that support the aims of value in health, i.e. the achievement of the outcomes that matter to people and the creation of a more sustainable healthcare system. These levers might be policy levers, financial levers or the realignment of organizational performance targets towards a much greater focus on actual patient outcomes. The importance of a national role in driving forward value-based healthcare cannot be overstated. Value-based healthcare leadership should foster the creation of the multidisciplinary network at a national level; it should join the dots at a system level and break down silos of thinking to ensure that all the elements of value-based healthcare described in this book are driven forward.

Value-based healthcare is a huge undertaking. It requires a seismic shift in culture and attitudes from all stakeholders in health. As we saw in chapter 3, we must make the revolution happen: creating the right organizational structures and implementing good policy are not enough. National and local value-based healthcare teams must – in parallel with working on implementation – continue to communicate and engage locally, regionally, nationally and internationally. This work should be relentless if we are to achieve better outcomes, equity and sustainability in healthcare.

Apprenticeship: passing the baton

Medicine is an apprenticeship. Doctors, nurses and allied healthcare professionals all have professional degrees, but none of us learns our trade until we start working directly with patients, guided and taught by our senior team members and mentors. Understanding the challenges of modern healthcare systems should now become an important part of both undergraduate and postgraduate curricula, and a lens needs to be focused on how to practice medicine that places importance on patient outcomes. However, unless senior clinicians model the way, formal education will not be sufficient within the timescales needed to change the way we deliver healthcare. This is why communication and engagement, and the constant giving of encouragement to each other as we undertake this challenging work, is so important. In Wales there is now a critical mass of clinical leaders applying the principles of value-based health-care in their own fields. Value-based healthcare has a life of its own, and that has given all of us in Wales hope that things can be better for patients, and we can regain joy and purpose in the practice of medicine.

Changing a healthcare system's culture towards one that is focused on outcomes and value enables a federated approach to creating value initiatives to emerge. In Wales there is still a long way to go to arrive at a point where we can say we have equitably improved outcomes and sustainability for the whole population, as we saw in the OECD data. What we can say is that we have improved outcomes for specific groups, and the culture has evolved to the extent that organizations and networks continue to grow and to drive this change from the grassroots.

I am unable to say how many successful value-based health-care interventions there currently are, and this inability is an encouraging sign of cultural shift. One great example is the work of Dr Mel Thomas and her colleagues in Lymphoedema Network Wales. In the box below you will find Dr Thomas's description of the work in her own words.

Driving value-based care in lymphoedema management: the Lymphoedema Wales Clinical Network model

The Lymphoedema Wales Clinical Network (LWCN) exemplifies a pioneering approach to value-based lymphoedema care across the life course. From its inception, LWCN has prioritized equity, sustainability, and outcome-driven service delivery

– minimizing waste, harm and variation. With lymphoedema prevalence now estimated at 7 per 1,000 people, these principles are more vital than ever. Central to LWCN's success is its commitment to patient self-management, viewed through a psychosocial lens that focuses on what matters most to each individual. In 2014, LWCN laid the groundwork for a responsive and comprehensive patient-reported outcome measure (PROM), culminating in the launch of LYMPROM© in 2020. This tool, now used across the UK and internationally, has also inspired the development of CELLUPROM© – the world's first cellulitis-specific PROM.

LYMPROM© is embedded in key pathways, including new patient referrals and patient-initiated follow-up, enabling PROM-led care that aligns clinical priorities with patient goals. For example, one patient's aspiration to resume caravan holidays became a shared goal, achieved through collaborative care, and improved lymphoedema management.

Since 2020, the National Cellulitis Improvement Programme has tackled the health and economic burden of cellulitis. With over 42,000 patients invited and 7,761 completing the programme, outcomes have dramatically improved: cellulitis episodes dropped from 8,232 to 280, hospital admissions from 4,329 to 53, and length of stay from 31,932 to 318 days. CELLUPROM© revealed fear of recurrence as a key concern – addressed through person-centred care, leading to measurable improvements in patient-reported outcomes.

LWCN's data-driven, person-focused model continues to set the standard for value-based lymphoedema care, demonstrating real-world impact at scale.

There is a very good reason why the work of Dr Thomas and her colleagues in Lymphoedema Network Wales has been so successful and enduring. Previously, outside of the clinical world, lymphoedema was a poorly understood condition that attracted no attention from decision makers within the system. By reaching out to other clinical disciplines, finance professionals, managers, academia and latterly the Welsh Value in Health Centre, Dr Thomas not only raised the profile of the condition but created momentum behind the achievement of better outcomes for patients living with this distressing condition. The progress achieved will endure beyond her tenure.

Leadership in pursuit of value-based healthcare

Of course, the golden thread running through all the successful work being done in value-based healthcare in Wales and around the world is leadership: passionate and principled professionals who hold a strong belief that things can and will be better for patients and the people taking care of them. Without these people – who believe that things can and should be better, who do not wait for permission but stand up and challenge the status quo – we will never see the radical changes to healthcare systems that are needed. We need people with a revolutionary mindset, just like those described throughout this book.

But leaders cannot work in isolation or hold onto plaudits for 'their' work too tightly. Value-based healthcare, radical healthcare system transformation, outcomes-focused care – whatever we prefer to call it – requires humble, boundary-spanning leaders. Leaders who are prepared to step outside their tribe and collaborate with those working in other disciplines to solve the challenges we face in health and in society as a whole. Leaders who, with humility and generosity, cede power and kudos to others. And leaders who, when the time comes, pass the baton on, for others to take the work forward.

Key lessons from chapter 8

Redesigning services requires system-wide collaboration

Value-based healthcare is not just a clinical responsibility. While clinicians are key, real transformation requires payers, policymakers, providers, and professionals from finance, digital and analytics to align.

Healthcare fragmentation is a major barrier. Especially in systems such as those in the United States, France, Germany and Australia, care remains too focused on hospitals due to disjointed pathways. Integrated care is the solution. Achieving seamless, person-centred care demands collaborative, multi-disciplinary work across all levels of the system.

Context is important

The principles of value-based healthcare are universal but must be applied with consideration given to the unique healthcare system and sociopolitical context of a region or country. Mandating or imposing externally developed blueprints for implementation are unlikely to be successful.

Implementation pitfalls to avoid

Do not lead with data collection without a purpose. Implementing PROMs or any other data collection without a clear change agenda risks disengagement and data misuse.

Cultural change is essential. Outcomes-focused care must be supported by a parallel shift in organizational mindset and strategy.

Avoid copy–paste models. Adapting value-based healthcare frameworks from other countries – not simply transplanting hem – is essential for success.

Build local and national capacity

Education is foundational. Organizations need a critical mass of people who understand value-based healthcare and are trained to implement it.

Multidisciplinary teams are vital. Practical implementation needs professionals with varied expertise: clinical, financial, digital and analytical professionals must work together if we are to find solutions that improve outcomes and create equitable, sustainable healthcare systems.

Internal and national teams play different roles. Local teams drive change on the ground; national centres align policy, infrastructure and levers, especially facilitating communities of practice to share learning and good practice.

Value-based healthcare is an ongoing apprenticeship

Formal training is not enough. Real learning happens in clinical practice, through mentorship and modelling by senior leaders.

Culture change needs champions. Constant communication, encouragement and visible examples of value-based healthcare in action sustain momentum.

Leadership makes the difference

Leadership is the golden thread in successful value-based healthcare stories. Effective leaders are boundary spanning. They reach beyond their disciplines, they share credit and they collaborate generously. Succession planning matters. Leadership in value-based healthcare requires humility to 'pass the baton' and let others carry the work forward.

Value-based healthcare is both a mindset and a method. It is not a plug-and-play model but a cultural and operational shift that requires leadership, humility and relentless collaboration across systems and professions. Without those who believe things can and should be better, we will never see the radical changes that are needed in healthcare.

About the author

Sally Lewis, the founder of Kintsugi International, is a distinguished leader in the field of value-based healthcare. With a remarkable career spanning 30 years as a general practitioner, medical leader and policy advisor, Sally has dedicated her career to transforming healthcare systems worldwide. She is recognized as a global pioneer in the implementation of value-based healthcare. She is now an international consultant on value-based healthcare system transformation and the Professor of Value in Health Management at Swansea University's value-based health and care academy.

As the former National Clinical Director for Value-Based and Prudent Healthcare in NHS Wales and the founder of the internationally recognized Welsh Value in Health Centre, she has pioneered the implementation of value-based healthcare, making substantial contributions to global healthcare improvements. Her work has been recognized by many institutions, including the World Economic Forum, Harvard Business School, Bertelsmann-Stiftung, the Organisation for Economic Co-operation and Development (OECD), HTAi and the Australian Healthcare and Hospitals Association. She is an international public speaker on health system transformation on the principles of value-based healthcare implementation.

Notes

Chapter 1

1 Bevan Commission. 2015. A prudent approach to health: prudent health principles (https://bevancommission.org/wp-content/uploads/2023/09/A-Prudent-Approach-to-Health-Prudent-Principles.pdf).

2 Well-being of Future Generations Act (Wales) 2015 (testimony of Welsh Government) (https://futuregenerations.wales/discover/about-future-generations-commissioner/future-generations-act-2015/).

3 A healthier Wales: long term plan for health and social care. 2018. Health and Social Care Strategy (https://gov.wales/healthier-wales-long-term-plan-health-and-social-care).

4 Bodenheimer, T., and Sinsky, C. 2014. From triple to quadruple aim: care of the patient requires care of the provider. *Annals of Family Medicine* 12(6): 573–76 (https://doi.org/10.1370/afm.1713).

5 Sackett, D. L., Rosenberg, W. M. C., Gray, J. A. M., Haynes, R. B., and Richardson, W. S. 1996. Evidence based medicine: what it is and what it isn't. *BMJ* 312(7023): 71–72 (https://doi.org/10.1136/BMJ.312.7023.71).

6 Slow Medicine: https://www.slowmedicine.it/.

7 *The BMJ*, 'Reducing overuse in healthcare': https://www.bmj.com/content/reducing-overuse-healthcare.

8 Fenning, S. J., Smith, G., and Calderwood, C. 2019. Realistic medicine: changing culture and practice in the delivery of health and social care. *Patient Education and Counselling* 102(10): 1751–55 (https://doi.org/ 10.1016/j.pec.2019.06.024).

9 Duncan, A. N., and Sayers, R. 2023. Getting it right first time: what have we learnt? *Surgery (Oxford)* 41(8): 489–94 (https://doi.org/10.1016/J.MPSUR.2023.05.002).

10 Elwyn, G., Frosch, D., Thomson, R., Joseph-Williams, N., Lloyd, A., Kinnersley, P., Cording, E., Tomson, D., Dodd, C., Rollnick, S.,

Edwards, A., and Barry, M. 2012. Shared decision making: a
model for clinical practice. *Journal of General Internal Medicine* 27:
1361–67 (https://doi.org/10.1007/s11606-012-2077-6).

11 Gawande, A. 2014. *Being Mortal: Medicine and What Matters in the
End*. New York: Metropolitan Books, Henry Holt and Company.

12 Amri, M., Siddiqi, A., O'Campo, P., Enright, T., and Di Ruggiero,
E. 2020. Underlying equity discourses of the World Health
Organization: a scoping review protocol. *Social Science Protocols* 3:
1–16 (https://doi.org/10.7565/ssp.2020.2812).

13 Groft, S. C., Posada, M., and Taruscio, D. 2021. Progress, challenges
and global approaches to rare diseases. *Acta Paediatrica* 110(10):
2711–16 (https://doi.org/10.1111/apa.15974).

14 Hart, J. T. 1971. The inverse care law. *The Lancet* 297(7696): 405–12.

15 Larsson, S., Clawson, J., Kellar, J., and Howard, R. 2022. *The Patient
Priority: Solve Health Care's Value Crisis by Measuring and Delivering
Outcomes That Matter to Patients*. McGraw Hill.

16 Wennberg, J. E. 2011. Time to tackle unwarranted variations in
practice. *BMJ* 342(7799): 687–90 (https://doi.org/10.1136/BMJ.
D1513).

17 Sackett *et al.* (1996), 'Evidence based medicine'.

18 Porter, M. E., and Teisberg, E. O. 2006. *Redefining Health Care:
Creating Value-based Competition on Results*. Google eBook
(https://books.google.com/books/about/Redefining_Health_Care.
html?id=cse2LOAndNIC).

19 Rolfson, O., Wissig, S., van Maasakkers, L., Stowell, C.,
Ackerman, I., Ayers, D., Barber, T., Benzakour, T., Bozic, K.,
Budhiparama, N., Caillouette, J., Conaghan, P. G., Dahlberg, L.,
Dunn, J., Grady-Benson, J., Ibrahim, S. A., Lewis, S., Malchau, H.,
Manzary, M., March, L., Nassif, N., Nelissen, R., Smith, N., and
Franklin, P. D. 2016. Defining an international standard set of
outcome measures for patients with hip or knee osteoarthritis:
consensus of the international consortium for health outcomes
measurement hip and knee osteoarthritis working group. *Arthritis
Care and Research* 68(11): 1631–39 (https://doi.org/10.1002/
acr.22868).

Chapter 2

1 ICHOM: https://www.ichom.org/.

2 Kotter, J. P. 1995. Leading change: why transformation efforts
fail. *Harvard Business Review* May–June (https://hbr.org/1995/05/
leading-change-why-transformation-efforts-fail-2).

3   European Commission: Directorate-General for Health and Food
    Safety. 2019. Defining value in 'value-based healthcare': report of
    the expert panel on effective ways of investing in health (EXPH).
    Publications Office (https://data.europa.eu/doi/10.2875/35471).

4   Gray, M., Wells, G., and Lagerberg, T. 2017. Optimising allocative
    value for populations. *Journal of the Royal Society of Medicine*
    110(4): 138–43 (https://doi.org/10.1177/0141076817698653).

5   Nuti, S., Vola, F., and Bonini, A. 2016. Making governance work
    in the health care sector: evidence from a 'natural experiment'
    in Italy. *Health Economics, Policy and Law* 11: 17–38 (https://doi.
    org/10.1017/S1744133115000067).

6   Salinas, J., Sprinkhuizen, S. M., Ackerson, T., Bernhardt, J.,
    Davie, C., George, M. G., Gething, S., Kelly, A. G., Lindsay, P.,
    Liu, L., Martins, S. C. O., Morgan, L., Norrving, B., Ribbers,
    G. M., Silver, F. L., Smith, E. E., Williams, L. S., and Schwamm,
    L. H. 2016. An international standard set of patient-centred
    outcome measures after stroke. *Stroke* 47(1): 180–86 (https://doi.
    org/10.1161/STROKEAHA.115.010898/-/DC1).

7   Burns, D. J. P., Arora, J., Okunade, O., Beltrame, J. F.,
    Bernardez-Pereira, S., Crespo-Leiro, M. G., Filippatos, G. S.,
    Hardman, S., Hoes, A. W., Hutchison, S., Jessup, M., Kinsella,
    T., Knapton, M., Lam, C. S. P., Masoudi, F. A., McIntyre, H.,
    Mindham, R., Morgan, L., Otterspoor, L., Parker, V., Persson, H. E.,
    Pinnock, C., Reid, C. M., Riley, J., Stevenson, L. W., and McDonagh,
    T. A. 2020. International Consortium for Health Outcomes
    Measurement (ICHOM): standardized patient-centred outcomes
    measurement set for heart failure patients. *Heart Failure* 8(3):
    212–22 (https://doi.org/10.1016/J.JCHF.2019.09.007).

8   MacKillop, E., and Sheard, S. 2018. Quantifying life: understanding
    the history of quality-adjusted life-years (QALYs). *Social
    Science & Medicine* 211, 359–66 (https://doi.org/10.1016/J.
    SOCSCIMED.2018.07.004).

9   Ernst, P., Saad, N., and Suissa, S. 2015. Inhaled corticosteroids in
    COPD: the clinical evidence. *European Respiratory Journal* 45(2):
    525–37 (https://doi.org/10.1183/09031936.00128914).

10 National Institute for Health and Care Excellence. 2018. Chronic
    obstructive pulmonary disease in over 16s: diagnosis and
    management. Guidelines, December, NICE (www.nice.org.uk/
    guidance/ng115).

11 Bazell, C., Alston, M., Pelizzari, P., and Sweatman, B. 2023. What
    are bundled payments and how can they be used by healthcare
    organizations? Milliman, 27 March (https://www.milliman.com/en/

insight/what-are-bundled-payments-and-how-can-they-be-used-by-healthcare-organizations).

12 Engels, N., Bos, W. J. W., de Bruijn, A., van Leeuwen, R., van der Meer, N. J. M., van Uden-Kraan, C. F., de Bey, P., and van der Nat, P. B. 2024. Santeon's lessons from a decade of implementing value-based health care. *NEJM Catalyst* 5(1) (https://doi.org/10.1056/CAT.23.0232).

13 Kaplan, R. S., and Anderson, S. R. 2004. Time-driven activity-based costing. *Harvard Business Review*, November (https://hbr.org/2004/11/time-driven-activity-based-costing).

14 Dias, A. G., Roberts, C. J., Lippa, J., Arora, J., Lundström, M., Rolfson, O., and Tonn, S. T. 2017. Benchmarking outcomes that matter most to patients: the Globe Programme. *European Medical Journal* 2(2): 42–49 (https://doi.org/10.33590/EMJ/10310677).

15 Welsh Government. n.d. Putting value at the centre of health and care in Wales (https://vbhc.nhs.wales/files/vbhc-national-action-plan/).

16 Welsh Government. 2019. Valuing our health: Chief Medical Officer for Wales annual report 2019. Report, May, Welsh Government (https://www.gov.wales/sites/default/files/publications/2019-05/valuing-our-health.pdf).

17 CEDAR – Centre for Healthcare Evaluation: https://cedar.nhs.wales/.

18 Welsh Value in Health Centre. n.d. Our strategy 2021–2024 (https://vbhc.nhs.wales/files/our-strategy-to-2024/).

Chapter 3

1   Kotter, J. P. 1995. Leading change: why transformation efforts fail. *Harvard Business Review* May–June (https://doi.org/10.1016/0029-1021(73)90084-4).

2   Sivers, D. 2010. The dancing man. YouTube, 11 February (https://bit.ly/4fuNsMq).

3   Gabe-Walters, M., and Thomas, M. 2021. Development of the lymphoedema patient reported outcome measure (LYMPROM). *British Journal of Nursing* 30(10): 592–98 (https://doi.org/10.12968/BJON.2021.30.10.592/FORMAT/EPUB).

4   Bacon, E., and Laing, H. 2024. A focus on value: evolving the heart failure service at Aneurin Bevan University Health Board in Wales, UK (part A). Case Study, The Case Centre (https://www.thecasecentre.org/products/view?id=200724).

5   NHS Wales Executive, 'NHS Wales cardiovascular atlas of variation': https://executive.nhs.wales/functions/networks-and-planning/cardiovascular/nhs-wales-cardiovascular-atlas-of-variation/.

6   Swansea University, 'Value-based health and care academy': https://www.swansea.ac.uk/som/vbhc-academy/.

7   Kotter, J. P. 1995. Leading change: why transformation efforts fail. *Harvard Business Review* May–June (https://doi.org/10.1016/0029-1021(73)90084-4).

8   Welsh Government. 2021. National clinical framework: a learning health and care system. Guidance Document, May, Welsh Government (https://www.gov.wales/national-clinical-framework-learning-health-and-care-system).

9   *BMJ*, 'Too much medicine': https://www.bmj.com/too-much-medicine.

10 Hardie, T., Horton, T., Thornton-Lee, N., Home, J., and Pereira, P. 2022. Developing learning health systems in the UK: priorities for action. Report, September, The Health Foundation, London (https://doi.org/10.37829/HF-2022-I06).

11 Larsson, S., Kellar, J., and Clawson, J. 2022. *Patient Priority: Solve Health Care's Value Crisis by Measuring and Delivering Outcomes That Matter to Patients*. McGraw Hill (https://www.ebooks.com/en-gb/book/210672764/the-patient-priority-solve-health-care-s-value-crisis-by-measuring-and-delivering-outcomes-that-matter-to-patients/stefan-larsson/).

12 Welsh Value in Health Centre, 'New video helps Welsh patients living with a chronic disease make their own diet choices': https://vbhc.nhs.wales/latest-news/latest-news/new-video-helps-welsh-patients-living-with-a-chronic-disease-make-their-own-diet-choices/.

13 OECD. 2025. Does healthcare deliver? Results from the patient-reported indicator surveys (PaRIS). Report, February, OECD Publishing, Paris (https://doi.org/10.1787/c8af05a5-en).

14 Welsh Value in Health Centre – YouTube: https://www.youtube.com/channel/UCoN7cyeJO3M3Hy-aKGg-1Iw.

Chapter 4

1   Ahmad, N., Ellins, J., Krelle, H., and Lawrie, M. 2014. Person-centred care: from ideas to action: bringing together the evidence

on shared decision making and self-management support. Report, October, The Health Foundation, London.

2   Elwyn, G., Edwards, A., and Thompson, R. (eds). 2016. *Shared Decision Making in Health Care*. Oxford University Press (https://doi.org/10.1093/acprof:oso/9780198723448.001.0001).

3   Brunet, M. 2020. *The GP Consultation Reimagined: A Tale of Two Houses*. Scion Publishing, Banbury.

4   Pereira Gray, D. J., Sidaway-Lee, K., White, E., Thorne, A., and Evans, P. H. 2018. Continuity of care with doctors: a matter of life and death? A systematic review of continuity of care and mortality. *BMJ Open* 8(6): Paper e021161 (https://doi.org/10.1136/bmjopen-2017-021161).

5   Dixon, A., Khachatryan, A., Wallace, A., Peckham, S., Boyce, T., and Gillam, S. 2011. Impact of quality and outcomes framework on health inequalities. Report, April, King's Fund (https://www.kingsfund.org.uk/insight-and-analysis/reports/impact-quality-outcomes-framework-health-inequalities).

6   Rudebeck, C. E. 2019. Relationship based care: how general practice developed and why it is undermined within contemporary healthcare systems. *Scandinavian Journal of Primary Health Care* 37(3): 335–44 (https://doi.org/10.1080/02813432.2019.1639909).

7   OECD. 2025. Does healthcare deliver? Results from the patient-reported indicator surveys (PaRIS). Report, February, OECD Publishing, Paris (https://doi.org/10.1787/c8af05a5-en).

8   European Medicines Agency, 'Real world data versus real world evidence': https://www.ema.europa.eu/en/about-us/how-we-work/data-regulation-big-data-other-sources/real-world-evidence.

9   NICE. 2021. Atrial fibrillation decision aid. Guidance, June, National Institute for Health and Care Excellence, London (https://www.nice.org.uk/guidance/NG196).

10 Dean, S., Mathers, J. M., Calvert, M., Kyte, D. G., Conroy, D., Folkard, A., Southworth, S., Murray, P. I., and Denniston, A. K. 2017. 'The patient is speaking': discovering the patient voice in ophthalmology. *British Journal of Ophthalmology* 101(6): 700–8 (https://doi.org/10.1136/bjophthalmol-2016-309955).

11 Nakanishi, E., and Takahashi, R. 2022. Side effects, contraindications, and drug–drug interactions in the use of antiparkinsonian drugs. In *NeuroPsychopharmacotherapy*,

pp. 2963–72. Springer International Publishing (https://doi.
org/10.1007/978-3-030-62059-2_218).

12 Greene, J., and Hibbard, J. H. 2012. Why does patient activation
matter? An examination of the relationships between patient
activation and health-related outcomes. *Journal of General Internal
Medicine* 27(5): 520–26 (https://doi.org/10.1007/s11606-011-1931-2).

Chapter 5

1 OECD. 2025. Does healthcare deliver? Results from the patient-
reported indicator surveys (PaRIS). Report, February, OECD
Publishing, Paris (https://doi.org/10.1787/c8af05a5-en).

2 Nano, J., Carinci, F., Okunade, O., Whittaker, S., Walbaum, M.,
Barnard-Kelly, K., Barthelmes, D., Benson, T., Calderon-Margalit,
R., Dennaoui, J., Fraser, S., Haig, R., Hernández-Jimenéz, S.,
Levitt, N., Mbanya, J. C., Naqvi, S., Peters, A. L., Peyrot, M.,
Prabhaharan, M., Pumerantz, A., Raposo, J., Santana, M., Schmitt,
A., Skovlund, S. E., Garcia-Ulloa, A. C., Wee, H.-L., Zaletel, J., and
Massi-Benedetti, M. 2020. A standard set of person-centred
outcomes for diabetes mellitus: results of an international and
unified approach. *Diabetic Medicine* 37(12): 2009–18 (https://doi.
org/10.1111/dme.14286).

3 Hoogendoorn, C. J., Shapira, A., Roy, J. F., Kane, N. S., and
Gonzalez, J. S. 2020. Diabetes distress and quality of life in adults
with diabetes. In *Behavioral Diabetes*, pp. 303–28. Springer (https://
doi.org/10.1007/978-3-030-33286-0_20).

4 Singapore Ministry of Health Agency for Care Effectiveness:
https://www.ace-hta.gov.sg/.

5 Waiyaya, E., De Sanctis, T., Njeri Wairimu, R., Otieno, M.,
Janssens, W., and Katuwal, S. 2022. A scalable mental health
intervention for women in Kenya. Policy Brief, September,
PharmAccess Foundation (https://www.pharmaccess.
org/wp-content/uploads/2022/09/Mental-Health-policy-
brief-02092022_2.pdf).

6 Healthy Outback Communities Western Queensland Primary
Health Network: https://www.healthyoutbackcommunities.com.
au/.

7 Hijry, H. 2024. Proposed model for NEOM city based on Internet
of Things (IoT) and MLC at ED system. In *2024 IEEE International
Conference on Prognostics and Health Management (ICPHM)*,
pp. 23–32 (https://doi.org/10.1109/ICPHM61352.2024.10627366).

8   Atkinson, C., Hughes, S., Richards, L., Sim, V. M., Phillips, J., John, I. J., and Yousef, Z. 2024. Palliation of heart failure: value-based supportive care. *BMJ Supportive and Palliative Care* 14(e1): e1225–e1233 (https://doi.org/10.1136/bmjspcare-2021-003378).

9   Akpan, A., Roberts, C., Bandeen-Roche, K., Batty, B., Bausewein, C., Bell, D., Bramley, D., Bynum, J., Cameron, I. D., Chen, L.-K., Ekdahl, A., Fertig, A., Gentry, T., Harkes, M., Haslehurst, D., Hope, J., Hurtado, D. R., Lyndon, H., Lynn, J., Martin, M., Isden, R., Mattace Raso, F., Shaibu, S., Shand, J., Sherrington, C., Sinha, S., Turner, G., De Vries, N., Jia-Chyi Yi, G., Young, J., and Banerjee, J. 2018. Standard set of health outcome measures for older persons. *BMC Geriatrics* 18(1): Paper 36 (https://doi.org/10.1186/s12877-017-0701-3).

Chapter 6

1   Campbell, B., Wilkinson, J., Marlow, M., and Sheldon, M. 2019. Generating evidence for new high-risk medical devices. *BMJ Surgery, Interventions, and Health Technologies* 1(1): Paper e000022 (https://doi.org/10.1136/bmjsit-2019-000022).

2   NHS Wales Health Collaborative. 2019. Cardiovascular atlas of variation. Report, March, NHS Wales Health Collaborative (https://performanceandimprovement.nhs.wales/functions/networks-and-planning/cardiovascular/cvn-docs/cardiovascularatlasofvariation-march2019-pdf/).

3   Eichler, H., Pignatti, F., Schwarzer-Daum, B., Hidalgo-Simon, A., Eichler, I., Arlett, P., Humphreys, A., Vamvakas, S., Brun, N., and Rasi, G. 2021. Randomized controlled trials versus real world evidence: neither magic nor myth. *Clinical Pharmacology and Therapeutics* 109(5): 1212–18 (https://doi.org/10.1002/cpt.2083).

4   Avşar, T. S., Elvidge, T., Hawksworth, C., Kenny, J., Németh, B., Callenbach, M., Ringkvist, J., and Dawoud, D. 2024. Linking reimbursement to patient benefits for advanced therapy medicinal products and other high-cost innovations: policy recommendations for outcomes-based agreements in Europe. *Value in Health* 27(11): 1497–1506 (https://doi.org/10.1016/j.jval.2024.07.007).

5   Skinner, B. F. 2019. *The Behavior of Organisms: An Experimental Analysis*. BF Skinner Foundation.

6   Larsson, S., Clawson, J., Keller, J., and Howard, R. 2022. *The Patient Priority: Solve Health Care's Value Crisis by Measuring and Delivering Outcomes That Matter to Patients*. McGraw Hill.

Chapter 7

1   Hookman, P., and Barkin, J. S. 2009. Clostridium diffcile associated infection, diarrhea and colitis. *World Journal of Gastroenterology* 15(13): Paper 1554 (https://doi.org/10.3748/wjg.15.1554).

2   HFMA, 'What is patient-level costing?': https://www.hfma.org.uk/healthcare-value-institute/what-is-PLICS.

3   Porter, M. E. 2010. What is value in health care? *New England Journal of Medicine* 363(26): 2477–81 (https://doi.org/10.1056/NEJMp1011024).

4   Dunstan, C., Huckle, D., Hosker, E., and Amer, S. 2024. Measuring performance in clinical outcomes: anaesthetics. *BJA Open* 12, 100332 (https://doi.org/10.1016/j.bjao.2024.100332).

5   Basch, E. 2017. Patient-reported outcomes: harnessing patients' voices to improve clinical care. *New England Journal of Medicine* 376(2): 105–8 (https://doi.org/10.1056/NEJMp1611252).

6   Akpan, A., Roberts, C., Bandeen-Roche, K., Batty, B., Bausewein, C., Bell, D., Bramley, D., Bynum, J., Cameron, I. D., Chen, L.-K., Ekdahl, A., Fertig, A., Gentry, T., Harkes, M., Haslehurst, D., Hope, J., Hurtado, D. R., Lyndon, H., Lynn, J., Martin, M., Isden, R., Mattace Raso, F., Shaibu, S., Shand, J., Sherrington, C., Sinha, S., Turner, G., De Vries, N., Jia-Chyi Yi, G., Young, J., and Banerjee, J. 2018. Standard set of health outcome measures for older persons. *BMC Geriatrics* 18(1): Paper 36 (https://doi.org/10.1186/s12877-017-0701-3).

7   Ayaz, M., Pasha, M. F., Alzahrani, M. Y., Budiarto, R., and Stiawan, D. 2021. The fast health interoperability resources (FHIR) standard: systematic literature review of implementations, applications, challenges and opportunities. *JMIR Medical Informatics* 9(7): Paper e21929 (https://doi.org/10.2196/21929).

8   Delussu, G., Frexia, F., Mascia, C., Sulis, A., Meloni, V., del Rio, M., and Lianas, L. 2024. A survey of openEHR clinical data repositories. *International Journal of Medical Informatics* 191: Paper 105591 (https://doi.org/10.1016/J.IJMEDINF.2024.105591).

9   Kamel Boulos, M. N., Brewer, A. C., Karimkhani, C., Buller, D. B., and Dellavalle, R. P. 2014. Mobile medical and health apps: state of the art, concerns, regulatory control and certification. *Online Journal of Public Health Informatics* 5(3): Paper e61275 (https://doi.org/10.5210/ojphi.v5i3.4814).

10 Mckenna, S. P., Wilburn, J., Thorsen, H., and Brodersen, J. 2012. Adapting patient-reported outcome measures for use in new

languages and cultures. In *Rasch Models in Health*, pp. 303–16. Wiley (https://doi.org/10.1002/9781118574454.ch16).

11 Nuti, S., Noto, G., Vola, F., and Vainieri, M. 2018. Let's play the patients music. *Management Decision* 56(10): 2252–72 (https://doi.org/10.1108/MD-09-2017-0907).

12 Vola, F., Benedetto, V., Vainieri, M., and Nuti, S. 2022. The Italian interregional performance evaluation system. *Research in Health Services and Regions* 1(1): Paper 10 (https://doi.org/10.1007/s43999-022-00010-6).

www.ingramcontent.com/pod-product-compliance
Lightning Source LLC
Chambersburg PA
CBHW041734200326
41518CB00020B/2587